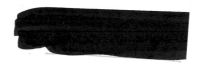

CW00458617

The Management of the Diabetic

To Rosemary and
Anne, Katherine, Christopher and David

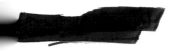

The Management
of the Diabetic Foot

Irwin Faris

MB BS (Melb), MD (Monash), FRACS

Senior Lecturer in Surgery, The University of Adelaide;
Senior Visiting Surgeon, Royal Adelaide and The Queen Elizabeth Hospitals,
Adelaide.
Formerly John Astor Fellow, The Middlesex Hospital Medical School;
Wellcome Clinical Research Fellow, Royal Postgraduate Medical School,
London.

Foreword by

L.P. LeQuesne

DM, MCh, FRCS, FRACS (Hon)

Professor of Surgery,
The Middlesex Hospital Medical School, London;
Deputy Vice-Chancellor and Dean of the Faculty of Medicine,
University of London.

CHURCHILL LIVINGSTONE
EDINBURGH LONDON MELBOURNE AND NEW YORK 1982

CHURCHILL LIVINGSTONE
Medical Division of Longman Group Limited

Distributed in the United States of America by
Churchill Livingstone Inc., 1560 Broadway, New
York, N.Y. 10036, and by associated companies,
branches and representatives throughout the world.

First published 1982
  Reprinted 1984
  Reprinted 1986

ISBN 0-443-02315-8

British Library Cataloguing in Publication Data
Faris, Irwin
    The Management of the diabetic foot.
    1. Diabetes — Complications and sequelae
    2. Foot — Diseases
    I. Title
616.4'62   RC660

Library of Congress Cataloging in Publication Data
Faris, Irwin, M.D.
    The management of the diabetic foot.
    Includes bibliographical references and index.
    1. Foot — Blood-vessels — Diseases — Treatment.
    2. Diabetes — Complications and sequelae.
    I. Title II. Title: Diabetic Foot. [DNLM:
    1. Diabetes mellitus — Complications. 2. Foot
      diseases — Etiology. 3. Foot diseases — Therapy.
    WK 835 F228m]
    RC951.F37   617'.585   82–4127
                                     AACR2

Produced by Longman Singapore Publishers Pte Ltd
Printed in Singapore

Foreword

Notwithstanding the fact that the fundamental defect affects carbohydrate metabolism, diabetes mellitus is a disease with widespread effects throughout the body, and the care of the diabetic patient may well comprise a multiplicity of problems, involving many organs and systems, notably the eyes, the kidneys, the blood vessels and the peripheral nerves. It is likely that with improved control of the underlying metabolic defect – a goal that seems within reach with various techniques currently under investigation – the incidence of these complications of diabetes mellitus will fall, and there can be no question that in the long term the goal to be achieved is their prevention rather than their management. None the less, at the present time it remains the case that these complications are an important cause of disability and real distress for many patients with this common disease, and their management constitutes an essential part of the care of many diabetics.

An important group amongst diabetic patients presenting problems due to these complications is formed by those with problems affecting the foot. Although not as common as some other complications, such as those affecting the eye, these are of particular importance to the patient as ultimately they may lead to the necessity for amputation of the foot or lower leg. This will result in grave disability if, as is tragically only too often the case, the patient's eyesight is also impaired. This group is also of great importance to the Health Services because of the long periods of hospital care that these patients may require. The foot complications are due to a variety of causes, notably arterial disease, peripheral neuropathy and skeletal deformity, often with sepsis complicating the picture. Probably because of this multiplicity of causative factors, their complications have tended to fall into a no-man's land between orthopaedic, vascular and general surgeons, diabetic physicians and chiropodists. As a result, they have not, in general, received the expert, detailed study they merit.

However, in recent years growing attention has been paid to the causes and management of the foot problems that beset diabetic patients, and the time is ripe for a book such as this to bring together our increasing understanding of this inter-related group of conditions. With a long-standing interest in these problems Mr Faris has himself carried out important studies into various aspects of the neuropathic complications. Furthermore, he is an experienced vascular surgeon. He is thus ideally equipped by the pattern of his clinical experience and by his combination of clinical and research expertise in the field, to master the interlocking factors that contribute to the totality of the 'diabetic foot'. In this admirably lucid book Mr Faris surveys the whole field related to our understanding and management of these problems. By bringing together in this single volume all the different aspects of problems which, although anatomically circumscribed in their clinical manifestations, are wide-ranging in the physiological and pathological disturbances involved, Mr Faris enables the whole problem of the 'diabetic foot' to be seen and comprehended in its entirety. As such this book is a much-needed addition to the bibliography of diabetes mellitus.

I have for many years been involved in the care of diabetic patients with foot problems, and for some time have felt that a book of this scope was needed. It is, therefore, a real privilege to be asked to write this foreword to this admirable book, which should help many clinicians, both physicians and surgeons, to a clearer understanding of these difficult problems, and thus help many patients to whom these complications of diabetes can be a great burden.

1982   L.P.LeQ.

Preface

The problem of the diabetic foot has been described by two eminent authorities in the following terms: 'one of the common major unsolved problems of clinical practice in the western world' (Eastcott, 1974)[1] and 'The annual costs of medical care for diabetes-related leg-vessel disease in this country (USA) probably exceeds $100 million' (West, 1978)[2]. Nor is the problem confined to people of Anglo-Saxon origin: many important contributions to our understanding have come from India and South Africa. Despite the frequency of the condition, the attendants of a diabetic patient with a foot lesion frequently experience feelings of confusion and pessimism. The confusion arises from the difficulty in understanding the pathological processes which are occurring and the pessimism from the gloomy prognosis which attends many of these patients.

This book does not provide easy solutions to either of these difficulties. The problems of assessment and management remain among the most challenging of those that are commonly seen in our hospitals and clinics. However, understanding can be improved by breaking the problem into its component parts. When this is done it is seen that the pathological processes involved are few. With regard to management, the greatest attention must be given to the prevention of lesions. If this fails additional treatment is required but there are only a small number of modalities about which knowledge is necessary. This book aims to provide information at a level which can be understood by anyone concerned in the care of these patients. Readers with more specialized interests may find that the references will guide them to more detailed information. It is the hope that the reader will come to understand the mechanisms of pathogenesis and the treatment available for these patients.

My interest in this subject was stimulated while working in Professor L. P. Le-Quesne's department at The Middlesex Hospital, London, and I am deeply indebted to him for his encouragement and his kindness in agreeing to write the foreword. I am also grateful to my colleagues in Adelaide for their help. Mr Adrian Burke, Professor John Ludbrook and Mr Glyn Jamieson and my wife have made many helpful comments on parts of the draft manuscript. Dr Philip Harding, Director of Endocrinology at the Royal Adelaide Hospital has provided the Appendix. Miss Jenny Ryan and Miss Ann Winter drew the line diagrams. The

[1]Eastcott H. H. G. 1974 Book Review. *British Journal of Surgery* 61: 928
[2]West K. M. 1978 *The epidemiology of diabetes and its vascular lesions*. Elsevier, New York ch 2

later stages of the manuscript were written while on study leave in Copenhagen in the Department of Clinical Physiology at Bispebjerg Hospital and I am most grateful to Dr N. A. Lassen for the facilities which he provided.

A number of colleagues have kindly allowed me to reproduce material. The patient whose X-rays are reproduced in Figures 3.7, 3.8 and 9.1 was under the care of Mr A. K. House and the illustrations are reproduced with his permission and that of Dr S. F. Yu. Figures 8.1, 8.3, 8.5, 8.6, 8.7 and 10.3 are reproduced with the permission of Professor LeQuesne. I am indebted to Mr W. C. Hutton and Springer Verlag for permission to reproduce Figure 6.6; to Dr P. Holstein and Munksgard, Copenhagen for Figure 9.5; and to Dr Lassen and W. B. Saunders & Co for Figure 9.6. Figure 7.1 is reproduced with the permission of the Medical Director, Royal Adelaide Hospital. Finally, my special thanks are due to Miss C. M. Anderson for her patient and efficient typing of the manuscript.

Adelaide, 1982

I. F.

Contents

1. A brief history of diabetes and its complications   1
2. Mechanisms for the development of foot lesions   4
3. Vascular disease   8
4. Neuropathy   25
5. Infection and wound healing   38
6. Mechanical factors   47
7. Prevention of major lesions   58
8. Clinical features of major lesions   71
9. Assessment of the patient with a foot lesion   80
10. Management   97
Appendix: Perioperative management of diabetes
         by P. E. Harding, MB, FRACP.   128
Index   129

1

A brief history of diabetes and its complications

Diabetes is one of many common diseases known from antiquity. A disease with polyuria is mentioned in the Ebers papyrus which includes Egyptian medical compilations dating from the second millenium B.C. In the middle of the second Christian century Aretaeus of Cappodocia used the Greek word for a syphon (διαβητηζ) to describe a disease in which water did not remain long in the body. The features included thirst, weight loss and polyuria. At about the same time Galen attributed this disease to the inability of the kidneys to retain water so that it passed through unchanged. The first account of sweet urine was reportedly given in India about 500 A.D. This preceded by more than 1000 years the account of Thomas Willis in 1675. In addition, it was recognized that there was a less harmful form of the disease in which the urine was tasteless.

In the second half of the eighteenth century, important advances were made. Robert Wyatt found a sugar-like substance in urine following evaporation. In the same period Frank classified the disease into two forms: *diabetes insipidus* (or spurious) in which there was no sugar in the urine or *diabetes mellitus* (or vera) in which the urine contained sugar.

The modern era can be said to have begun with the work of John Rollo who in 1798 concluded that diabetes was a disease of the stomach which resulted in the abnormal transformation of vegetable nutritive matter into sugar. He prescribed a treatment regimen of carbohydrate restriction which soon fell from favour because it may well have been worse than the disease. In the nineteenth century, progress was rapid. McGregor and Magendie separately found sugar both in the blood of diabetics and, in small quantities, in blood from normal subjects. More detailed knowledge of the metabolism of sugar had to await the studies of Claude Bernard.

Early suggestions of the involvement of the pancreas in diabetes followed the 1885 observation that the administration of phloridzin to an animal was followed by glycosuria. The classic experiments of pancreatic ablation were performed shortly afterwards by Von Mering and Minkowski although they had been attempted 40 years earlier by Bouchardat. The link between the pancreas and diabetes was unknown but the disease could be prevented by transplanting a fragment of the pancreas. In 1892 Lepine proposed that diabetes was due to the absence of a glycolytic ferment in the pancreatic juice but pathological confirmation of the link was not achieved until Opie in 1900 demonstrated the connection between disease of the islets of Langerhans and diabetes. Sharpey-Schafer concluded that the islands of Langerhans must secrete a substance which regulates carbohydrate metabolism and in 1916 proposed the name of insulin for this hypothetical substance. The discovery of insulin in 1921 ranks with the discovery of penicillin and streptomycin in the benefit it conferred to sufferers of an incurable lethal disease. The book by Wrenshall et al (1962) gives a vivid account of this dramatic period. Following the introduction of insulin, when death in coma became a less frequent outcome of the disease, attention began to be turned to the longer-term complications and it was soon recognized that deaths from vascular disease had become more common.

The association between diabetes and symptoms in the limbs was first recognized by John Rollo (1798). His patient had pains and paraesthesiae 'lumbago and sciatica in so great a degree as to be nearly deprived of the use of the lower limbs'. Indeed before 1850 the frequency of neurological changes in diabetics led to suggestions that neuropathy was the cause of diabetes. In the period between 1850 and 1870 both gangrene and plantar ulcers were recognized as complications of diabetes. In 1888 Hunt collected 72 cases of diabetic gangrene and concluded that 'gangrene in diabetes is something more than a coincidence'. During the last 30 years of the century there were rapid advances in understanding of neurological complications. Absence of tendon reflexes, abnormalities of sweating and motor paralysis were described and pathological examination revealed degenerative changes in the peripheral nerve and the dorsal columns of the spinal cord.

The association between foot ulceration, neuropathy and vascular disease was first recorded by Pryce (1887):

'The patient was a 56–year old man who had symptoms of diabetes for 18 months. For three months he had noticed ulceration on the regions of the first right metatarsophalangeal joint and the fifth left metatarsophalangeal joint. There was decreased sensation of the lower one third of the legs and feet and the knee jerks were absent. The legs were livid and cold. Death in coma occurred four days later. At autopsy degenerative changes were noted in the dorsal and lumbar parts of the spinal cord and in the peripheral nerves. There was atheromatous disease of the posterior tibial arteries and of its smallest branches'.

In 1893 he reported two further cases. In each case there was marked atheroma of the posterior tibial artery and 'blocking up of smaller microscopic blood vessels'. His conclusions were that, while neuritis in young diabetics might be due to a specific toxic poison, in older subjects it was due to vascular disease. The idea that vascular disease was the cause of neuritis, ulceration and gangrene was for the next 50 years the dominant influence both on thoughts on the pathogenesis of foot lesions and in plans of treatment.

The emphasis on vascular disease as a cause of foot lesions meant that until quite recently major amputations were performed frequently for small areas of gangrene. In the pre-antibiotic era the mortality in these patients was very high and many patients were treated by their physicians for long periods perhaps because they feared that major amputation was the only alternative. However, some surgeons were able to report occasional successes with local amputation but clear indications for local or major amputation were not established for much of this period. Thus the success of local treatment in selected cases had been demonstrated but it is clear that these were the fortunate patients: inability to control the diabetes and spreading sepsis caused the death of many.

In the period 1920–1950 arterial disease was believed to be the dominant factor in the development of foot lesions. The hypothesis that disease of the microscopic blood vessels might be the cause of several of the major complications of diabetes was put forward in 1941 when the association between retinopathy, neuropathy and nephropathy was noted and the suggestion made that the common factor was disease of the blood vessels. This view was reinforced by reports in 1959 in which changes in the vessels in amputated limbs and in small nerve biopsies were described (see Ch. 4 for details). However, observations of a dissociation between vascular disease and neuropathy gave rise to two important changes in opinion. They were that:

1. metabolic rather than vascular factors might cause neuropathy, and
2. neuropathy, independent of vascular disease, might cause foot lesions.

This latter view was most clearly recognized by Oakley et al, who in 1956 described the classification of foot lesions which is widely used to the present time.

REFERENCES

Oakley W, Catterall R C F, Martin M M 1956 Aetiology and management of lesions of the feet in diabetics. British Medical Journal 2: 953–957
Pryce T D 1887 A case of perforating ulcers of both feet with diabetes and ataxic symptoms. Lancet 2: 11–12
Rollo J 1798 Cases of the diabetes mellitus, 2nd Edn. C Dilly, London, p 260
Wrenshall G A, Hetenyi G, Feasby W R, Marcus A 1962 The story of insulin. The Bodley Head, London

2

Mechanisms for the development of foot lesions

The classification of Oakley et al (1956) was a major step forward in our understanding of the causes of foot problems in diabetic patients. They classified the causes as: (1) Ischaemia, (2) Neuropathy, (3) Infection (4) Combined.

This outline is the basis of current classifications which have been presented in a more detailed form (see Du Plessis 1970).

The complications of diabetes predispose to the development of foot lesions. These complications, the onset of which is unpredictable, are largely irreversible. Thus when they occur the foot becomes vulnerable. However patients may live for many years and die from another manifestation of the vascular disease, e.g. nephropathy or myocardial infarction, without ever having a significant foot infection or ulcer. This is because these patients have avoided the precipitating factors, the most important of which is mechanical trauma. Minor wounds or infections in a foot with normal sensation and normal blood supply are recognized by the pain they cause hence treated early and heal rapidly. In the ischaemic, anaesthetic foot a small lesion may progress because it is not recognized and the source of injury not removed. Impairment of the blood supply may result in delayed healing. Infection is an important aggravating factor which may cause extensive tissue damage.

In this chapter an outline of the pathogenic mechanisms will be given. Detailed discussion of their occurrence and importance is given in the subsequent chapters. The factors responsible for the development of foot problems in diabetics can be classified as:

Predisposing Factors
    Vascular disease
    Neuropathy
    Liability to infection
Precipitating Factors
    Physical injury
        mechanical trauma
        heat
    Infection

PREDISPOSING FACTORS

Vascular disease (Ch. 3)

Atherosclerosis. This may cause ischaemic foot lesions in diabetics, just as it does in non-diabetics, and is the most important factor in about half the patients seen in developed countries. If the blood supply to the foot is reduced sufficiently, minor wounds will not heal and there may be ischaemic pain at rest. Neuropathy frequently coexists but this is a mixed blessing. On the one hand, the patient is spared the pain of an ischaemic foot, but on the other hand, tissue damage and infection may progress unnoticed. Spread of infection, especially with anaerobic organisms, is potentiated by the ischaemia of the tissues and the consequent inability of the blood supply to increase sufficiently to effectively combat local infection.

Calcification of arteries. This is an indicator of a prolonged diabetic metabolic disturbance but there is no evidence that it is an important factor in the development of foot problems.

Microangiopathy. The role of disease of arterioles and capillaries is still controversial. If the disease were sufficiently widespread, local blood flow might be reduced to such a degree that ischaemic lesions could develop and extend as outlined above. However there is no convincing evidence that microvascular changes are severe enough to act in this way. Nor is there good evidence that they potentiate the effects of atherosclerosis. It is possible that micro-angiopathy has no significant role in the development of foot lesions (see p. 34).

Neuropathy (Ch. 4)

The major components are:

a. Loss of perception of pain. This and ischaemia are the two most important factors in the development of severe foot lesions.

b. Paralysis of the small muscles of the foot. This results in clawing of the toes and a decreased effective load-bearing area under the forefoot. Thus abnormal forces may affect both the deformed toes and the area of the metatarsal heads.

c. Autonomic neuropathy. This might potentiate the development of lesions by (i) failure of reflex dilatation in response to local injury; (ii) abnormal vasoconstriction in response to cold.

Impaired perception of pain means that small injuries go unrecognized and thus progress before diagnosis. This often causes loss of tissue, but there is no direct evidence that these factors aid the development of infection.

Infection

Decreased resistance to infection may be both a precipitating and aggravating factor. The possible mechanisms are discussed in Chapter 5 and include:

a. Abnormal cellular and humoral response to inflammation. This may be potentiated by impairment of the blood supply and dysfunction of the autonomic nervous system.

b. Decreased efficiency of the process of repair, the most important component of which is collagen formation. Once infection has occurred the presence of ischaemia may facilitate spread as outlined above.

PRECIPITATING FACTORS

Despite the presence of the predisposing factors an uninjured foot may not develop serious problems. However physical trauma is a potent cause of trouble (see Ch. 6).

a. A puncture wound, e.g. from ingrowing toenail, will allow the entry of bacteria and infection may result. In addition, if there is severe ischaemia of the tissues progressing necrosis may follow.

b. Localized pressure, e.g. from tight shoes, may cause ischaemic necrosis.

c. Repeated mechanical trauma, e.g. from walking, may cause inflammation and subsequent necrosis.

d. Heat, e.g. from a hot water bottle, may burn the skin if there is reduced perception of temperature and pain sensation.

Some of the interactions of these predisposing and precipitating factors are shown in the diagram (Fig. 2.1). The underlying principle is that the predisposing factors reduce the ability to cope with minor injuries which progress to form major lesions. The exception to this rule is that severe vascular disease may cause gangrene in the absence of mechanical trauma.

This concept of predisposing and precipitating factors has important implications for the management of diabetic patients. In general the vascular disease and neuropathy cannot be reversed (although their development may be delayed –

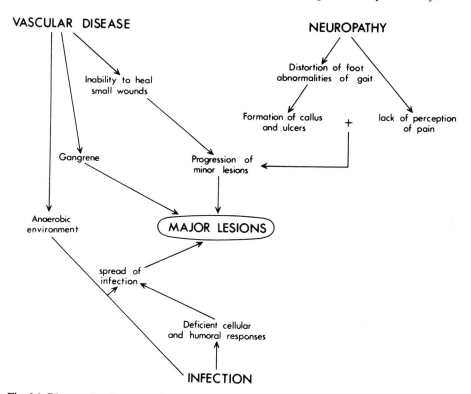

Fig. 2.1 Diagram showing some of the mechanisms by which the major predisposing factors aid the development of major lesions

see p. 59). However the precipitating factors may be regarded as being preventable and thus the rigorous avoidance of physical trauma would prevent the development of most of the problems which occupy so much of the resources of our hospitals and clinics. This preventative approach is emphasized in Chapter 7. Unfortunately this approach often fails and the latter part of the book (Ch. 9 and 10) describes the methods of assessment and treatment for the salvage of these limbs.

REFERENCES

Oakley W, Catterall R C F, Martin M M 1956 Aetiology and management of lesions of the feet in diabetics. British Medical Journal 2: 953–957
DuPlessis D J 1970 Lesions on the feet in patients with diabetes mellitus. South African Journal of Surgery 8: 29–46

3

Vascular disease

INTRODUCTION

Disease of blood vessels is a major cause of complications in diabetics. It may affect both capillaries, the smallest blood vessels across which nutrient exchange occurs in the tissues, and the largest arteries, the aorta and its branches. Obstruction of the larger vessels may cause the complications of stroke or myocardial infarction while disease of the smaller vessels causes loss of vision (diabetes is the commonest cause of blindness in many Western communities) and kidney failure. The following sections give accounts of the types of arterial disease, their prevalence and effects.

Disease is commonly described as affecting large or small vessels. The unqualified use of the term 'small vessel disease' has often made understanding of this subject very difficult, particularly when considering possible effects on the foot. The term may be given several meanings:

a. Disease of arterioles and capillaries (Syn. 'microangiopathy'). Small vessel disease in this context has often been inappropriately blamed as a cause of foot changes which were primarily due to neuropathy.

b. Disease of arteries in the calf. Severe disease of these vessels usually leads to amputation but reconstructive surgery can sometimes be employed.

c. If the arteries of the calf and arterioles are involved, are the arteries in between, i.e. the metatarsal and digital arteries, affected by arterial disease?

The term 'small vessel disease' should be abandoned unless the context of its use makes perfectly clear the sorts of vessels being described.

ATHEROSCLEROSIS

Atherosclerosis is the commonest cause of death in many Western societies. It may be defined as a degenerative vascular disease affecting principally the tunica intima of arteries and composed of fibrous and/or fatty change. Ulceration and secondary thrombosis commonly occur. It has been believed for many years that this condition occurred more frequently and with greater severity in diabetics. There has been controversy about the truth of this belief and this has only recently been satisfactorily resolved. (For detailed references see West 1978). There are several lines of evidence which support the view that there is an increased occurrence of vascular disease in diabetics.

Community surveys

The best evidence has come from prospective studies which have involved large samples of patients from single communities. These studies have been carried out in many regions (North America, Scandinavia, Eastern Europe, South Africa, Great Britain, Australia) with similar results. They show that both the prevalence and incidence of vascular disease is increased in diabetics. The study carried out in Framingham, Massachusetts, demonstrated that diabetes was an independent risk factor in the development of coronary heart disease, the incidence of cardiovascular disease (coronary, cerebral and peripheral) was increased, and the risk of death from cardiovascular disease was increased more in women than in men (Kannel and McGee 1979). This latter finding is of particular interest because it shows that the diabetic woman loses the relative immunity from vascular disease that non-diabetic women enjoy. This risk also applies to people who are hyperglycaemic but not frankly diabetic. Recently prepared criteria for the diagnosis of diabetes (National Diabetes Data Group 1979) include a category of impaired glucose tolerance. In the Whitehall study (Fuller et al 1980) subjects with blood glucose levels of ≥ 5.37 mmol/l had a coronary heart disease mortality at $7\frac{1}{2}$ years of the same order as that of known diabetics and twice that of those subjects with lower blood glucose levels. However this group of patients with impaired glucose tolerance was immune from the microvascular complications. Another approach has been to study prevalence of glucose intolerance in patients with symptomatic arterial disease. Wahlberg (1966) and Epstein (1967) have demonstrated that abnormalities of glucose tolerance occur more frequently than normal in patients with either coronary or peripheral vascular disease. One problem has been to determine if the observed abnormalities in glucose tolerance resulted from an episode of, for example, myocardial infarction but it has been shown that hyperglycaemia occurs in patients with coronary or peripheral arterial disease who do not have infarction or gangrene.

A further difficulty with these studies has been that the methods used for the diagnosis of arterial disease, particularly in the limbs, have been very insensitive. Marinelli et al (1979) have used non-invasive techniques for assessing the presence of arterial disease in a large prospective study of diabetics. They found that one-third of the patients without a history of intermittent claudication had evidence of arterial disease on testing. One-fifth of the subjects with normal physical findings had abnormal results to these tests. Clearly these methods provide a more sensitive means of diagnosing subclinical atherosclerosis in the leg.

Autopsy evidence

Shortly after the discovery of insulin, it was noted that many deaths in diabetic patients occurred from arterial disease. The evidence from autopsy studies (e.g. Bell 1950) which showed that diabetics frequently died of vascular disease has been criticized because of the difficulties in ensuring that the sample studied were representative (clearly patients undergoing autopsy are a specially selected sample) and in describing a high prevalence of one common disease in the presence of another. However the more recent autopsy evidence suggests that patients with diabetes have an increased risk of developing atherosclerosis (Robertson and Strong 1968).

Mechanisms

The theory of atherogenesis which is at present the most popular invokes as the cause proliferation of smooth muscle cells secondary to injury to the endothelium. The injury may be mechanical, e.g. hypertension, or chemical, e.g. hyperlipidaemia. This is followed by the accumulation of lipid and other extracellular components in the artery wall. The early changes may be reversible but the persistence of various risk factors, e.g. hyperlipidaemia, causes many lesions to progress. The mechanisms by which diabetes causes the accelerated development of atherosclerosis are not certain although many possibilities have been investigated and the topic has been reviewed recently by Ganda (1980).

Blood lipids

Raised values of triglycerides and cholesterol in the blood have been reported but the epidemiological evidence suggested that the concentrations were only marginally raised in treated diabetics. Much recent attention has been given to the possible protective role of high density lipoproteins (HDL), high concentrations of which give some protection against atherosclerosis. Several studies have shown that adult-onset diabetics have depressed HDL levels (Gordon et al 1977) although this might not apply to all sub-groups of diabetics (Reckless et al 1978 and Beach et al 1979).

Hypertension

Reports on the frequency of hypertension in diabetics vary in their conclusions. In most populations hypertension is more frequent in diabetics and this may contribute to the incidence of vascular disease but it is not the major cause of the increase (Jarrett and Keen 1975).

Hyperglycaemia

This has been shown to be an independent risk factor for the development of atherosclerosis in the Framingham and Busselton (WA) community studies. There is evidence from prevalence studies that there is a range of risks between groups with normal, borderline and clearly abnormal glucose metabolism. The possible mechanisms include impairment of vessel wall metabolism or nutrition, changes in coagulation, or osmotic effects. Hyperglycaemia may also have a direct stimulatory effect on the smooth muscle cell.

Hyperinsulism

The demonstration of an association between hyperglycaemia and vascular disease does not prove cause and effect. In addition there are several studies which suggest that control of the blood glucose does not decrease the risk of vascular disease and there are varying opinions on the relative importance of age and duration of diabetes on the development of vascular disease. Stout (1979) has suggested that a common factor in the development of atherosclerosis in adult-onset diabetics may be hyperinsulism and he has proposed several mechanisms by which inappropriate circulating insulin levels might facilitate atherogenesis.

Haematological factors

These are also discussed in the section on the cause of microangiopathy. Platelets release a substance, as yet unidentified, which is a potent stimulator of the proliferation of smooth muscle cells. Further, an area of endothelial damage causes platelet adhesion and aggregation, so that a self-potentiating process may be set up. The observation of increased platelet adhesiveness (see p. 20) provides a mechanism by which the process of atherogenesis might be enhanced in diabetics.

Humoral factors
The increased levels of growth hormone which are present in diabetics may accelerate the proliferation of smooth muscle cells. The increased concentrations of catecholamines which can be found in many diabetics may have the same effect.

Morphology and distribution
The macroscopic features of streaks and plaques of atheroma are indistinguishable in diabetics and non-diabetics but there is good evidence that the distribution of the disease is different.

In the leg the distribution of atherosclerosis has been studied by arteriography and the examination of amputation specimens. In non-diabetics the common patterns of disease are as follows:

Occlusion of the femoral artery
This is the most common lesion and characteristically starts at the region of the hiatus in the adductor magnus muscle where the femoral artery passes close to the femur. Extension of the occlusion to involve the whole length of the femoral artery is common.

Stenosis or occlusion of the aorta and/or iliac arteries
This may occur at any level from the origin of the renal arteries from the aorta to the inguinal ligament. Stenosis of the iliac arteries may be difficult to see on arteriograms taken in a single anteroposterior plane because the disease commonly forms a plaque along the posterior wall of the iliac artery.

Stenosis of the profunda femoris artery
This vessel, which is the major source of blood for the thigh muscles, is often affected by atheroma which causes narrowing at its origin. Such narrowing can be demonstrated in about 20% of patients with leg ischaemia. In a patient with obstruction of the femoral artery, this stenosis is sometimes treated instead of performing a bypass operation. More commonly it is corrected as part of an aorto-femoral reconstruction.

Diffuse disease
In addition to the patterns described, atherosclerosis may cause any combination of stenosis or occlusion of the arteries between the aorta and the ankle.

In diabetics the frequencies of the various patterns is different. Most seriously, the diabetic more frequently has multiple occlusions of the popliteal artery and its branches (Strandness et al 1964). (Figs. 3.1–3.4). This is important because it limits the application of reconstructive arterial surgery. There is relative sparing of the more proximal vessels: the iliac arteries are seldom occluded and the femor-

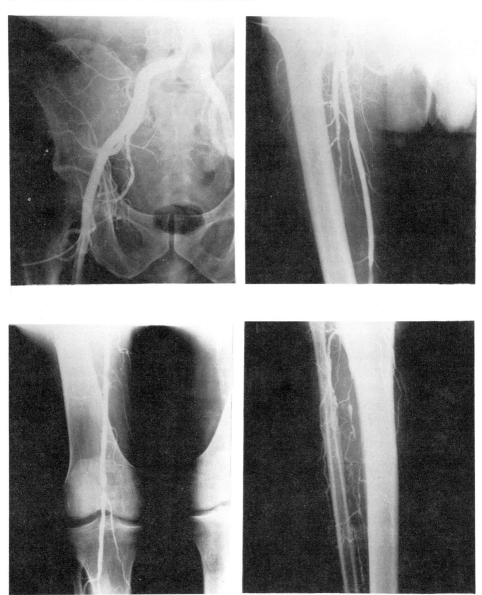

Figs. 3.1–3.4 Arteriogram showing the typical pattern of atherosclerosis associated with diabetes. The iliac arteries (3.1) and the upper part of the femoral artery (3.2) are patent. In the popliteal artery (3.3) there is a stenosing plaque of atheroma at the level of the intercondylar notch of the femur. The arteries of the calf (3.4) are very severely diseased. There is no possibility of improving the circulation by performing arterial surgery in such a limb.

al vessels often show irregular narrowings without occlusion. The more distal parts of the profunda femoris artery are also more commonly narrowed in diabetics. Thus in addition to the risk of developing arterial disease as in non-diabetics, the diabetic may develop a pattern of atherosclerosis affecting the leg arteries which carries a serious threat to the survival of the limb. It must be pointed out that not all studies have agreed with this view. The report of Strandness et al (1964) has been the most convincing, although other authors have found that there were no clear differences in the distribution and severity of atherosclerosis in amputated limbs (Goldenberg et al 1959; Conrad 1967). This may be because limbs which require amputation, whatever the cause, are likely to have severely diseased arteries.

Disease in the arteries of the foot has seldom been studied. There are several possible reasons for this including the difficulty of performing arteriography on the foot arteries and the inability to treat disease of these vessels. However if the tendency for arterial occlusion to affect the distal vessels is extended from the calf to the foot, this might have important implications for the healing in local areas of injury and might predispose to the spread of necrosis. Foot arteriography has shown that there may be hypervascularity and appearances suggesting microaneurysm formation.

Histological disease appeared as a uniform, although often asymmetrical, thickening of the tunica intima (Ferrier 1967) (Figs. 3.5–3.6). This contrasted with the lumpy appearance of atheromatous plaques in larger arteries. The diseased intima comprised a loose collagen network with pale ground substance and few nuclei. It did not stain with periodic acid-Schiff stain and did not contain elastic fibres. These changes were qualitatively similar in both diabetics and non-diabetics. The metatarsal arteries were, however, more often obstructed in diabetics. The nature of this disease is unknown but it is important because it demonstrates that arterial disease is contiguous from the aorta to the capillaries.

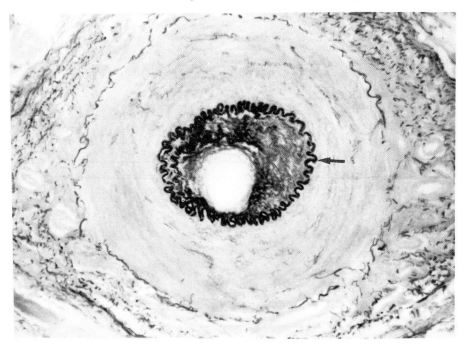

Figs. 3.5–3.6 Disease in small arteries

Fig. 3.5 The internal elastic lamina (arrow) encloses an eccentrically thickened tunica intima.

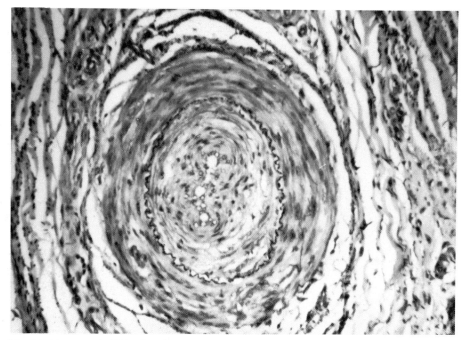

Fig. 3.6 Almost total obliteration of the lumen

CALCIFICATION OF ARTERIES

Calcification of the tunica media of muscular arteries is a common feature of long-standing diabetes, which is the commonest cause of these changes. Arterial calcification may result from deposition of calcium salts either in atheromatous plaques of the tunica intima, e.g. in the wall of an aortic aneurysm, or in the tunica media. Calcification in the tunica intima, which is common in atherosclerosis, has an irregular lumpy appearance on radiographs. In contrast calcification of the tunica media may be distinguishable because of its relatively regular, fine, speckled appearance (Fig. 3.7–3.8). In addition medial calcification commonly affects the vessels of the foot, which are seldom affected by atherosclerosis.

Several studies have demonstrated that medial calcification is more common in diabetics. Its frequency has been related to age, male sex and duration of diabetes in those aged less than 50 years. Neubauer (1971) made the interesting observation that calcification of the vessels of non-diabetics was related to higher levels of blood glucose following a glucose load. This suggests that hyperglycaemia has a direct role in the development of this condition and in this regard it is similar to atherosclerosis.

The effect of calcified vessels on the blood supply to the foot remains uncertain. It has been demonstrated that arterial calcification was associated with a reduction in the peak blood flow which is an index of the capacity of the circulation to increase. This alone would probably have only a minor effect on the blood supply to the foot. It has also been demonstrated that advanced vascular calcification was associated with narrowing or occlusion arising in the tunica intima. On

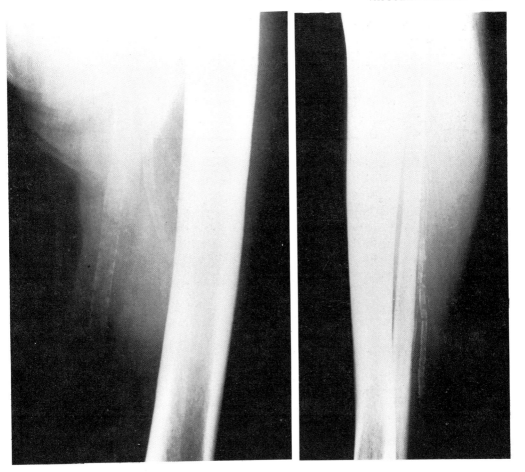

Figs. 3.7–3.8 Radiograph of thigh (3.7) and calf (3.8) showing very extensive calcification of large arteries. In the thigh the superficial and deep femoral arteries can be clearly identified. The fine regular pattern suggests that the calcification is in the tunica media

the other hand, the tunica intima may be relatively unaffected despite major deposits of calcium in the tunica media (see Fig. 3.9).

One important practical point is that calcification of the tunica media makes the wall of the artery difficult to compress so that measurement of the blood pressure by external compression of an artery will be less accurate. This phenomenon is well recognized but there is no reliable information about the frequency with which it occurs.

MICROANGIOPATHY

Two of the major causes of morbidity in diabetics, namely retinopathy and nephropathy, have been known for many years to be due to microvascular disease. An hypothesis that disease of the microscopic blood vessels might be the cause of the major complications was suggested by Dry and Hines (1941) who

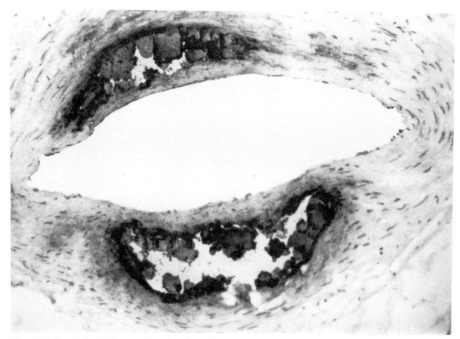

Figs. 3.9 Arterial calcification. Section through a muscular artery showing large plaques of calcification. The tunica intima is normal.

noted the clinical association between retinopathy, neuropathy and nephropathy and suggested that the common factor between them was disease of the small blood vessels. This reinforced the assumption that small vessel disease was important in the development of foot lesions as well.

Two reports in 1959 mark the beginning of modern research into the morphology and function of small vessels in diabetes. Goldenberg et al (1959) described in the small vessels of amputated limbs changes which they believed to be characteristic of diabetes. Fagerberg (1959) studied the small vessels in biopsy specimens from the sural nerve and considered that the changes which he saw were the cause of the neuropathy. The changes which are typical, if not pathognomonic, of diabetes can be divided into two histological groups.

Thickening of capillary basement membranes (Fig. 3.10)
When seen with the light microscope the appearances are of focal thickenings of the vessel wall. The staining reactions of these areas indicate the presence of glycoprotein. On electron microscopy, laminar thickening of the capillary basement membrane is seen and this is accompanied by changes in the nuclei of the perivascular cells. These changes have a patchy distribution and are believed to have a common origin with renal and retinal vascular disease.

In the limbs, these changes have been seen in the skin, muscle and nerves. Much research has been carried out on the identification of these changes because of the important role they play in the development of complications of diabetes. The time at which they develop has aroused much controversy. This began with the report that basement membrane thickening in skeletal muscle capillaries was

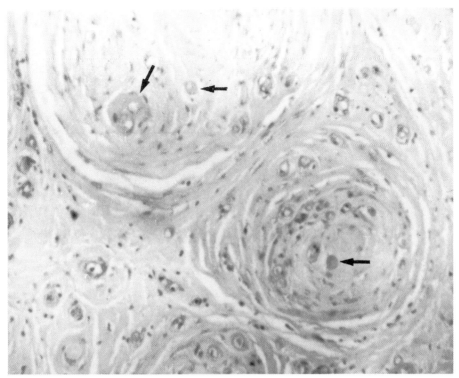

Fig. 3.10 Microangiopathy. PAS stain (X330). Section of a digital nerve from a toe. There are several capillaries (arrows) showing marked thickening of the basement membrane

present in patients who were genetically likely to develop diabetes and in patients with latent diabetes. It was suggested that these changes might be genetically determined. However, subsequent workers have been unable to confirm these findings and much of the subsequent disagreement has hinged on the precise techniques used in preparing and examining the speicmens. A majority view would now be that capillary basement membrane thickening follows, rather than precedes, the development of the metabolic derangement of diabetes (see Williamson 1979 for summary of arguments). Although these changes are characteristic of diabetes they are not exclusive to it because identical changes have been seen in a small proportion of specimens from non-diabetics.

Proliferative changes in arterioles and arteries

These findings include:

a. enlargement and proliferation of endothelial cells which might result in occlusion of the vessels.

b. concentric rings of periodic acid-Schiff positive staining material between which were enlarged endothelial cells.

c. single and intact internal elastic lamina.

d. normal tunica media.

In the initial report of Goldenberg et al (1959) these changes were described in vessels up to the size of the digital arteries and, like the capillary basement membrane thickening, they can be seen in some specimens from non-diabetics. They have been identified in many tissues from the limbs including skin, muscle, nerve and vasa vasorum. There is some doubt if these changes represent a specific form of vascular disease or if they are merely reactive, for example, obliterative changes in vessels whose capillary beds have been reduced in size.

Cause of microangiopathy

These morbid anatomical changes are the end result of metabolic disturbances which have continued for a prolonged period; e.g. the first signs of capillary basement membrane thickening in the kidney are not detectable until 18 months after the onset of diabetes. Much research has been carried out into the mechanisms whereby microangiopathy develops. It is possible to fit many of the observations into a reasonably coherent scheme although the details would not be universally agreed.

A number of abnormalities of vessel function and morphology can be detected early in diabetes. To these has been given the name 'functional microangiopathy'. The changes can be seen in young diabetics as abnormal vascular patterns in the mucosa of the cheek and alveolus and in the nailfold vessels. In the eye the retinal venules are dilated and there is perivascular oedema which suggests that there has been an increased exudation of large molecules through the vessel wall. These changes may be reversible and are not associated with definite histological abnormalities although irreversible changes develop more rapidly in the conjunctival vessels of diabetics than in normal subjects.

Functional changes may also be found in vessels in other parts of the body. There are several abnormalities of renal function which are detectable in early diabetes. There is an increase of glomerular filtration rate and an increase in the filtration fraction. This is probably explained by an increased permeability of glomerular capillaries which allows a greater loss of large molecules. In addition the kidneys of newly diagnosed diabetics are larger than normal. All of these changes can be reversed by restoring good control of the diabetes.

Evidence of vascular dysfunction is not confined to the eye and the kidney. In the limbs an increased blood flow can be shown to involve both muscle and subcutaneous adipose tissue. There is, in addition, evidence of a widespread leakiness of the capillaries which can be demonstrated as an increased rate of loss of labelled albumin from the blood.

From the observations described above it seems that the two major initial changes are:

    a. venular dilatation

    b. increased capillary permeability

On the basis of these observations, Ditzel has developed an hypothesis to explain their possible progression to organic microvascular disease (see Editorial, British Medical Journal (1977) for summary; Ditzel (1980) for details). The major element of this hypothesis is that tissue hypoxia would provide an explanation for the changes described and may be the initiating factor in the development of microangiopathy.

The functional changes described: vasodilation and increased capillary permeability, could be explained as a response to local hypoxia. This might result from a reduction in oxygen delivery to the tissues or an increased demand for oxygen. The former is probably the more important although an increased metabolic rate can be demonstrated in diabetics and this falls following the administration of insulin. At the same time the local vasodilation also decreases. There is considerable evidence to suggest that oxygen delivery to the tissues is reduced. The oxygen dissociation curve (Fig. 3.11) may be shifted to the left in diabetic patients. This shift means that for a given oxygen tension the percent saturation is higher i.e. more oxygen remains bound to the haemoglobin molecule therefore less is available to the tissues. Such a shift can be demonstrated acutely following both the administration of insulin and the treatment of ketoacidosis and may result in a significant reduction in the amount of oxygen available to the tissues at these times.

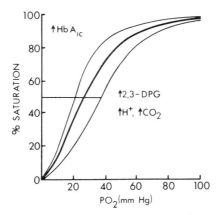

Fig. 3.11 Effect of increased concentrations of HbA$_{Ic}$, 2, 3-DPG, H$^+$ and CO$_2$ on the oxygen dissociation curve.

There are several factors which might cause this shift. One of the important regulators of oxygen release by the haemoglobin molecule is 2, 3-diphosphoglycerate (2, 3-DPG). This is a byproduct of glucose metabolism which reduces the affinity of haemoglobin for oxygen. The concentration in the red cells of 2, 3-DPG falls during the treatment of ketosis and this may worsen the local hypoxia. This probably occurs because insulin administration decreases the concentration of plasma inorganic phosphate and this inhibits 2, 3-DPG formation. In addition there may be increased amounts of haemoglobin A$_{Ic}$ (HbA$_{Ic}$) which has a greater avidity for oxygen and therefore also shifts the haemoglobin dissociation curve to the left. HbA$_{Ic}$ is believed to be formed by the non-enzymic addition of glucose to the end of the beta chain of the haemoglobin molecule (see p. 50 for more details). However it has been pointed out (Koenig and Cerami 1980) that mutant haemoglobin with a much greater affinity for oxygen is not associated with clinical vascular disease.

If hypoxia is prolonged, venular and capillary dilation may be followed by increased permeability of the vessel wall to protein. The protein which leaks represents most of the types of plasma proteins. This protein may be deposited in the vessel wall and it is postulated that this may initiate the histological changes. In addition to the mechanisms discussed above there are a number of observable changes in the blood which might impair blood flow through the smallest blood vessels.

Platelets

Several aspects of platelet function have been demonstrated to be abnormal in diabetics (Bern 1978). In each case the changes favour the development of thrombi.

a. Increased platelet adhesiveness has been demonstrated in platelets from diabetics. This may be dependent on increased activity in the plasma of the von Willebrand factor which is produced by endothelial cells.

b. Increased platelet aggregation. Once platelets have stuck to an area of endothelium, aggregation and the release to active substances from the platelets can occur. A number of studies have demonstrated that platelet aggregation induced by adenosine diphosphate, adrenaline and collagen is enhanced in diabetics. These changes may be reversed by aspirin. There is also evidence that the normal balance between thromboxane and prostacyclin activity is upset and this may influence platelet aggregation.

c. Other reported abnormalities related to blood clotting include reduced survival of both platelets and fibrinogen in diabetics.

While there is no direct evidence that these platelet abnormalities cause microangiopathy they are most commonly found in patients with the worst clinical microangiopathy. It is known that factors released from platelets caused enhanced endothelial permeability and proliferation of smooth muscle cells. Both these actions could be associated with the accelerated development of arterial disease (see also p. 11).

Red cells

The effect of changes in HbA_{Ic} and 2, 3-DPG in the red cells have been mentioned above. Other changes in the red cells include a greater rigidity, which probably means that they pass less readily through the smallest capillaries and a greater tendency to aggregate due to changes in plasma protein.

Plasma

Changes occur in the concentration of many of the plasma proteins. The groups most affected are those which characteristically increase in response to acute stress (actue-phase reactants). The concentrations are raised in a number of acute and chronic conditions, including diabetes even if patients with obvious acute causes for a rise are excluded. These changes are usually associated with a fall in serum albumin. In diabetics they are most marked in patients with severe microangiopathy.

Rises in plasma protein concentration are associated with increased plasma viscosity. The same proteins which increase viscosity will enhance the aggregation of red cells. Both these factors will tend to reduce blood flow through small blood vessels. There is also reduced activity of the fibrinolytic systems in the plasma and this will reduce the clearance of small amounts of fibrin which are deposited. It has been demonstrated that aggressive treatment of the diabetes reduces both the viscosity and the plasma fibrinogen levels (Paisley et al 1980).

The small blood vessels throughout the body are all exposed to these potentially damaging actions but the area most severely affected varies between patients. Careful histological examination has revealed abnormalities in capillaries and arterioles in many areas of the body and the clinical association between retinopathy and nephropathy has been recognized for many years. This has been confirmed by more recent studies which have recorded that half the deaths in patients with retinopathy were due to uraemia; the prognosis for vision was worse in patients with proteinuria and, in a separate study, all patients dying of uraemia had retinopathy. Reports on the association between microangiopathy and neuropathy vary in their conclusions although many longstanding diabetics will have microangiopathy and neuropathy as well as atherosclerotic vascular disease. On the other hand others have found no relationship between retinopathy and other manifestations of arterial disease.

Finally, to demonstrate the differences in pathogenesis between microangiopathy and atherosclerosis, it has been shown that while smoking was the best predictor for the development of intermittent claudication in the Framingham study, West et al (1980) could detect no relationship between smoking and microangiopathy.

There are many observations of abnormalities of metabolism which it is beyond the scope of this account to describe in detail. These include:

1. alterations in the activity of enzymes which attach carbohydrate to basement membrane proteins;

2. cellular function defects, e.g. changes to leucocyte function (see Ch. 5), alterations in the activity of lysosomal enzymes;

3. an alternative metabolic pathway for fructose synthesis which results in the accumulation of sorbitol. This may be important as a cause of neuropathy (see Ch. 4);

4. hormonal effects. An increased capillary fragility can be related to high levels of circulating growth hormone, while glucagon is probably important in maintaining hyperglycaemia.

A summary of the factors which may be important in the development of microangiopathy can be seen in Figure 3.12.

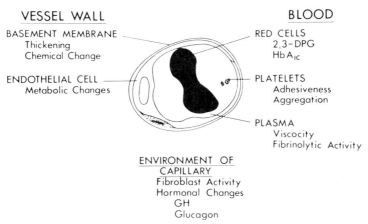

Fig. 3.12 Diagram showing some of the factors in the environment of a capillary which might be responsible for changes in its wall.

CLINICAL EFFECTS

Atherosclerosis

From the discussion of the occurrence of atherosclerosis in the diabetic leg, it can be deduced that diabetics are liable to the same consequences of impairment of the blood supply to the leg as non-diabetics. Thus diabetics may develop intermittent claudication which will manifest the same signs and require the same treatment as non-diabetics. If the occlusion is more severe, rest pain or gangrene may occur and again the clinical features and principles of treatment are identical in both diabetics and non-diabetics. However, the treatment may be more difficult in patients with diabetes because of the presence of atherosclerosis in the calf vessels (see p. 11 for detailed discussion).

Atherosclerotic occlusion is the major problem in about half the patients who present with foot ulcers or gangrene in Western communities which have large populations of maturity onset diabetics. In clinics seeing many young patients or in developing countries, atherosclerosis is less common as a cause of foot lesions.

Small vessel disease

The question of whether the microvascular changes are important in causing foot lesions is one of the unresolved problems in diabetes. This question may be considered in two parts.

Arteriolar and capillary disease

There have been several studies which have tried to assess the importance of these changes in the development of foot lesions. Moore and Frew (1965) found a strong association between the presence of foot lesions and the finding of proliferative changes in skin vessels. Conversely, Stary (1966) believed from his study of amputation specimens that the changes in the larger and medium sized arteries were sufficient to cause the skin necrosis seen. Similarly, Banson and Lacy (1964) found that lesions of small vessels were no more serious in diabetics with gangrene than in non-diabetics. Du Plessis (1970) found capillary changes in 50% of his patients with lesions, although he did not provide any information about their frequency in control subjects. In my own series microangiopathy can be found in about half the patients with foot ulcers. It is difficult to see how this patchy change in the smallest blood vessels could be responsible for large areas of necrosis. Nielsen (1973) found no cases with proliferative changes, and capillary changes in only 4 out of 15 diabetics with foot ulcers. He concluded that the microangiopathy did not cause the lesions. The evidence from these studies supports the conclusion that changes in capillaries and arterioles are probably not responsible for the development of ulcers and gangrene in diabetics.

Digital and metatarsal arteries

This is not usually considered to be an important factor but there are several lines of evidence which suggest an association between disease at this level and the development of foot lesions. If segmental blood pressures are measured, it is found that diabetics have a greater fall in pressure between ankle and toe than non-diabetics (Nielsen et al 1973). This observation has been extended with the report (Faris 1975) that larger gradients occur in those diabetics who develop foot ulcers and gangrene and this observation is independent of the presence of atherosclerosis in the leg (see Fig. 3.13). The pathological changes, which probably explain these observations, have been recorded by Ferrier (1967) and described above.

The diagnosis of vascular disease in patients with foot lesions is discussed in Chapter 9.

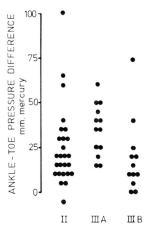

Fig. 3.13 Ankle-toe pressure gradient in three groups of feet. Left (II) Diabetics without foot ulcers. Centre (IIIA) Foot with an ulcer. Right (IIIB) Non-ulcerated foot of patient with ulcer. (See Chapter 9 for discussion of the method)

REFERENCES

Banson B B, Lacy P E 1964 Diabetic microangiopathy in human toes. American Journal of Pathology 45: 41–58
Beach K W, Brunzell J D, Conquest L L, Strandness D E 1979 The correlation of arteriosclerosis obliterans with lipoproteins in insulin-dependent and non-insulin-dependent diabetes. Diabetes 28: 836–840
Bell E T 1950 A postmortem study of 1214 diabetic subjects with special reference to the vascular lesions. Proceedings of the American Diabetes Association 10: 62–82
Bern M M 1978 Platelet functions in diabetes mellitus. Diabetes 27: 342–350
Conrad M C 1967 Large and small artery occlusion in diabetics and non-diabetics with severe vascular disease. Circulation 36: 83–91
Ditzel J 1980 Affinity hypoxia as a pathogenic factor of microangiopathy with particular reference to diabetic retinopathy. Acta endocrinologia 94: Suppl 39–55
Dry T J, Hines E A 1941 The role of diabetes in the development of degenerative vascular disease with special reference to the evidence of retinitis and peripheral neuritis. Annals of Internal Medicine 14: 1893–1902
Du Plessis D J 1970 Lesions on the feet in patients with diabetes mellitus. South African Journal of Surgery 8: 29–46
Editorial: Pathogenesis of Diabetic Microangiopathy. British Medical Journal 1977 1: 1555–1556
Epstein F H 1967 Hyperglycaemia: a risk factor in coronary heart disease. Circulation 36: 609–619
Fagerberg S – E 1959 Diabetic neuropathy. Acta medica Scandanavica Supp. 345: 1–80
Faris I 1975 Small and large vessel disease in the development of foot lesions in diabetics. Diabetologia 11: 249–253
Ferrier T M 1967 Comparative study of arterial disease in amputated lower limbs from diabetics and non-diabetics. Medical Journal of Australia 1: 5–11
Fuller R H, Shipley M J, Rose G, Jarrett R J, Keen H 1980 Coronary heart disease risk and impaired glucose tolerance. Lancet 1: 1373–1376

Ganda O P 1980 Pathogenesis of macrovascular disease in the human diabetic. Diabetes 29: 931–942

Goldenberg S, Alex M, Joshi R A, Blumenthal H 1959 Non-atheromatous peripheral vascular disease of the lower extremity in diabetes mellitus. Diabetes 8: 261–273

Gordon T, Castelli S P, Hjortland M C, Kannell W B, Dawber T R 1977 High density lipoprotein as a protective factor against coronary heart disease: the Framingham study. American Journal of Medicine 62: 707–714

Jarrett R G, Keen H 1975 Complications of diabetes. Edward Arnold, London

Kannel W B, McGee D L 1979 Diabetes and cardiovascular risk factors: the Framington study. Circulation 59: 8–13

Koenig R J, Cerami A 1980 Haemoglobin A_{Ic} and diabetes mellitus. Annual Review of Medicine 31: 29–34

Marinelli M R, Beach K W, Glass M J, Primozich J F, Strandness D E 1979 Noninvasive testing vs clinical evaluation of arterial disease. Journal of the American Medical Association 241: 2031–2034

Moore J M, Frew I D O 1965 Peripheral vascular lesions in diabetes mellitus. British Medical Journal 2: 19–23

National Diabetes Data Group 1979 Classification and diagnosis of diabetes mellitus and other categories of glucose intolerance. Diabetes 28: 1039–1057

Neubauer B 1971 A quantitative study of peripheral arterial calcification and glucose tolerance in elderly diabetics and non-diabetics. Diabetologia 7: 409–413

Nielsen P E 1973 Does diabetic microangiopathy cause development of gangrene? Scandinavian Journal of Clinical and Laboratory Investigation 31: Suppl 128: 229–234

Paisley R B, Harkness J, Hartog M, Chadwick T 1980 The effect of improvement in diabetic control on plasma and whole blood viscosity. Diabetologia 19: 345–349

Reckless J P D, Betteridge D J, Wu P, Payne B, Galton D J 1978 High-density and low-density lipoproteins and prevalence of vascular disease in diabetes mellitus. British Medical Journal 1: 883–886

Robertson E B, Strong J P 1968 Atherosclerosis in persons with hypertension and diabetes mellitus. Laboratory Investigation 18: 538–551

Stary H C 1966 Disease of small blood vessels in diabetes mellitus. American Journal of the Medical Sciences 252: 357–374

Stout R W 1979 Diabetes and atherosclerosis – the role of insulin. Diabetologia 16: 141–150

Strandness D E, Priest R E, Gibbons G E 1964 Combined clinical and pathologic study of diabetic and non-diabetic peripheral arterial disease. Diabetes 13: 366–372

Wahlberg F 1966 Intravenous glucose tolerance in myocardial infarction, angina pectoris and intermittent claudication. Acta medica Scandanavica 180: Suppl 453

West K M 1978 Epidemiology of diabetes and its vascular lesions. Elsevier, New York, ch. 10

West K M, Erdreich L S, Stober J A 1980 A detailed study or risk factors for retinopathy and nephropathy in diabetes. Diabetes 29: 501–508

Williamson J R, Kilo C 1979 A common sense approach resolves the basement membrane controversy in the NIH Pima Indian study. Diabetologia 17: 129–131

4

Neuropathy

INTRODUCTION

Impairment of nerve conduction is an important and frequent complication of diabetes. All types of fibres are involved so that motor, sensory and autonomic functions are affected. Minor degrees of impairment can be detected clinically in about one third of adult diabetics although nerve conduction studies will be abnormal in a greater number of patients. The changes in nerve function may be detectable at the time of diagnosis of the diabetes and tend to be gradually progressive, although improvement can occur with treatment and more rapid deterioration can be recognized to follow periods when the diabetes has been poorly controlled.

Neuropathy is an important cause of symptoms in diabetics whether they are related to the limbs or to the viscera, e.g. postural hypotension, impotence. However, ignorance of the neuropathy does not protect the patient from complications and this is particularly important in the foot, because patients with impaired sensation in the foot are at risk to the complications of neuropathy, whether or not they are aware of its presence. Neuropathy remains one of the major factors leading to the development of foot lesions in diabetics.

AETIOLOGY AND PATHOLOGY

The development of neuropathy was one of the early complications of diabetes to be recognized. Indeed, so common was neuropathy that it was suggested that neuropathy was the cause of the diabetes. Neuropathy was almost universally believed to be due to vascular disease until the report of Jordan (1936) who noted that not all his patients with trophic ulcers had arteriosclerosis. Since that time there has been the advancement of alternative hypotheses for the development of neuropathy. A recent review of the possible causes has been given by Clements (1979).

Vascular disease

There are two mechanisms by which vascular disease might cause lesions of nerves. They are (1) ischaemia caused by occlusion of vessels and (2) altered permeability of capillaries causing osmotic and metabolic derangements. The long history of vascular occlusion as a putative cause has been mentioned above.

However this idea has been challenged on several grounds:

a. The poor correlation between clinical and histological evidence of neuropathy on the one hand and demonstrable vascular disease on the other.

b. Neuropathy may improve with control of diabetes but there is no evidence that vascular disease improves.

c. In patients with severely ischaemic limbs, there may be very little evidence on clinical, electrophysiological or histological grounds of significant neuropathy.

There was a renewal of interest in vascular disease as a cause of neuropathy following the demonstration by Fagerberg (1959) of microvascular changes in sural nerve biopsies from diabetic subjects, but it is now generally agreed that arteriolar changes are not sufficiently widespread to account for the neuropathy.

A more plausible hypothesis rests on the possibility that increased capillary permeability to protein, which is a feature of diabetic microangiopathy in other sites, might either allow access to the nerve fibres of toxins (of which there is no definite evidence) or cause oedema and subsequent impairment of nutrition of the nerve. This idea, for which there is some experimental support (Jakobsen 1978), might also explain the fluctuations in the course of the condition which occur clinically. There is general agreement that vascular occlusion is the cause of one of the groups of neural lesions in diabetics. In patients with cranial nerve lesions and with severe, proximal motor neuropathy, there have been clear demonstrations of microscopic infarcts of the nerve associated with vascular thrombosis (Raff et al 1968).

Metabolic causes

There is much clinical and experimental evidence of an association between diabetic metabolic abnormalities and impaired nerve function. Examples include worsening of neuropathy which may follow periods when the diabetic control has been bad, the amelioration which may follow the achievement of good control, and the observation that in experimental diabetes functional alterations are present before demonstrable structural changes.

The description of segmental demyelination (Thomas & Lascelles 1966) as the dominant histological feature of diabetic neuropathy led to the idea that abnormalities of Schwann-cell function might be the cause of neuropathy. The observed improvement in the condition might result from remyelination which allowed nerve conduction. A number of mechanisms which might impair myelin production have been described. These include synthesis of abnormal myelin and increased activity of the polyol pathway which converts glucose to fructose. The latter abnormality might result in the accumulation of metabolites (e.g. sorbitol) which damage the Schwann cells and thus produce demyelination. The details of this mechanism are still the subject of considerable research.

An alternative explanation for the observed segmental demyelination is that it is secondary to a primary lesion in the axon. It is claimed that axonal damage occurs early in the disease and may be independent of Schwann cell damage. The evidence, which is largely based on animal models and is supported by both histological and electrophysiological studies, suggests that axonal damage is the first manifestation of diabetic neuropathy. The search for biochemical explanations at present centres on disturbances of axonal transport and the metabolism of myo-inositol which is found in high concentrations in normal nerves. It is of interest to note that Behse et al (1977) concluded, from a combined electrophysiological and histopathological study, that the processes of axonal degeneration and Schwann-cell changes proceeded independently of each other. This suggests that both processes may be important in the development of neuropathy. Currently it is considered that metabolic factors are more important than vascular disease in the development of neuropathy except in those cases which can be attributed to nerve infarction i.e. lesions of cranial and major peripheral nerves.

The characteristic histological finding in the peripheral nerves is of segmental demyelination. Single fibre studies have shown abnormal variation in the distance between adjacent nodes of Ranvier and these changes have been interpreted as indicating that subsequent remyelination has occurred. In addition there is loss of axons from nerves. It is suggested that loss of small fibres is greater than loss of larger fibres. Histological changes of degeneration have been described in the dorsal columns of the spinal cord and in the anterior horn cells. Changes in spinal nerve roots have been associated with spinal cord disease.

The histological changes in the autonomic nervous system have been less well studied. Quantitative studies (Low et al 1975) demonstrated that the myelinated fibre density was reduced in the splanchnic nerve of diabetics and teased fibre preparations showed that segmental demyelination and remyelination occurred as in the peripheral nerves. Some evidence of axonal degeneration was seen. In the sympathetic ganglia there was segmental loss of myelin and axonal degeneration of neurones in rami communicantes. The presence of cytoplasmic vacuoles in the nerve cells and of giant degenerative neurones have also been described. The vacuoles have been shown to be in the endoplasmic reticulum and to extend into dendritic processes (Duchen et al 1980). These changes are, however, occasionally found in patients without autonomic neuropathy and also in non-diabetics. Examination of the visceral nerve plexus of various parts of the gastrointestinal and genito-urinary systems has not produced a clear pattern of abnormalities. There has been one report of histological evidence of denervation of small blood vessels.

A variety of electrophysiological abnormalities can be demonstrated in these patients. Sensory nerve conduction abnormalities are the most consistent indicator of subclinical neuropathy (Thomas & Eliasson, 1975). There is decreased conduction velocity, and decreased amplitude and increased temporal dispersion of sensory action potentials, e.g. in the sural nerve. There is a widespread slowing of motor nerve conduction which increases with the duration of diabetes and this can be shown to vary with the control of the diabetes and to improve with treatment. In severer cases it may be impossible to demonstrate action potentials in the muscles of the foot (Harrison & Faris 1976).

CLINICAL FEATURES

The symptoms and signs of neuropathy may be related to somatic or autonomic nerve function. There may be a variety of syndromes which range from an insidious onset of irreversible neuropathy to the acute development of symptoms which recover with treatment. The following quotation from Colby (1965) illustrates the diversity of features:

'There is no diabetic neurologic syndrome, but rather a heterogeneous array of mononeuropathies, polyneuropathies, myelopathies and possibly encephalopathies, which vary in type, nature of onset, relationship to diabetic control, severity, prognosis and susceptibility to various therapeutic programs. The vagaries of diabetic neurologic disorders are so numerous that their recital leads to discouraging confusion.'

Despite this warning some attempt at classification is necessary in order to help understanding.

Somatic neuropathy

The commonest manifestation of diabetic neuropathy is a mild, distal, polyneuropathy. It is usually symmetrical and predominantly affects sensory fibres. The earliest detectable signs are absence of the ankle reflex and diminished perception of vibration at the ankle. At this stage the patient is usually unaware of any abnormality. There is dispute if these signs are significant or if they merely represent the changes of ageing. Mayne (1965) found that symptoms and signs of neuropathy were more common at all ages in a group of diabetic subjects although in his non-diabetic group ankle reflexes were impaired in one third of patients older than 50 and vibration sense at the ankle was impaired in two-thirds of patients aged 70 or older. A reasonable interpretation is that diabetes accelerates these age-associated changes.

The neuropathy may progress so that a glove-and-stocking type of peripheral neuropathy may be evident. In addition to the loss of ankle reflexes and of vibration sense at the ankle, there is decreased perception of light touch and pinprick in the toes and feet. In severer cases, these changes can extend to the leg. Once there has been loss of pain sensation, a critical phase of the disease has been reached because the anaesthetic foot is liable to suffer injuries which pass unrecognized. The neuropathy is usually slowly progressive and is not influenced by treatment. Some patients have a sub-acute onset of symptoms of neuropathy. This deterioration is often associated with a period of poor control of the diabetes or may be present at diagnosis of diabetes in middle-aged patients. When adequate control is achieved substantial improvement can occur. In these patients there may be pain in the foot which is often just a dull ache but which can have a deep burning character and may be worse at night. Pain with these characteristics may be difficult to distinguish from ischaemic rest pain (see Ch. 9). The signs are usually symmetrical and involve all modalities of sensation. Symptoms in the upper limb are seldom present although abnormalities of nerve conduction can be readily demonstrated by special testing.

A few patients develop signs of severe proximal muscle weakness and wasting. The muscles are usually painful, but there is little or no sensory loss. This 'diabetic amyotrophy' is usually easily distinguishable from the distal neuropathy. Complete resolution is usual. The pelvic girdle and thigh are most affected, with the quadriceps femoris muscle being especially involved. Occasionally the changes affect the shoulder girdle.

Major nerve lesions

There may be a loss of function of one or more major peripheral or cranial nerves. In most patients there is a gradual development of symptoms but occasionally the onset is rapid, and in these patients the onset is often preceded by a period during which it was recognized that the control of the diabetes was poor. The peripheral nerves most commonly affected are the median, ulnar and common peroneal nerves. The dominant upper limb is more often affected and this suggests that mechanical factors are important.

Several histological studies have demonstrated nerve infarcts in these patients and it is believed that these lesions are the result of nerve ischaemia (see section on Pathology). This notion is supported by the observation that in patients with mononeuropathy there are usually only minor degrees of somatic or autonomic neuropathy present (Fraser et al 1979), suggesting that the lesion results from a discrete episode rather than being a localised worsening of generalized changes. Cranial nerve lesions most commonly involve the oculomotor, abducent and facial nerves. These are usually acute in onset (over a period of days) and resolve spontaneously.

Autonomic neuropathy

Symptoms attributable to autonomic neuropathy have been described for many years as part of the diabetic syndrome but in the last ten years there has been a great increase in interest in this subject. The development of various tests which have been able to provide objective evidence of abnormality has allowed the demonstration of autonomic neuropathy in increasing numbers of diabetics and its incidence probably parallels that of somatic neuropathy. Impairment of autonomic function has been demonstrated in all sites where testing has been possible, and may be responsible for many of the symptoms of diabetes. Changes affecting the cardiovascular system have been the most intensively studied and the whole subject has been reviewed recently (Clarke et al 1979).

In general the autonomic neuropathy occurs at the same time as somatic neuropathy and both may be present at the time of diagnosis of diabetes (Fraser et al 1977). The detection of the changes of autonomic neuropathy may be of prognostic importance. In a small series (Ewing et al 1976) more than half the patients with symptomatic autonomic neuropathy and abnormal cardiovascular reflexes had died within 2½ years. This does not mean that the deaths were due to autonomic neuropathy although there are several mechanisms by which the effects of autonomic neuropathy might lead to the death of the patient, e.g. painless myocardial infarction (Lancet 1978), unawareness of hypoglycaemia and abnormalities of the control of ventilation. Table 4.1 lists the various manifestations of autonomic neuropathy which may occur. This chapter will consider in detail the peripheral circulatory changes because of their possible relevance to the development of foot ulcers.

Vasomotor and thermoregulatory changes

Abnormalities of the neural control of the vessels in the limbs were among the first manifestations of autonomic neuropathy to be studied. The limb vessels have an important role in the regulation of body temperature in addition to their func-

Table 4.1 Manifestations of autonomic neuropathy

1. Heart (Clarke et al 1979)
   a. Raised resting heart rate
   b. Postural hypotension
   c. Lack of beat-to-beat heart rate variation
   d. Abnormal baroreceptor responses (Bennett et al 1980)
   e. Painless myocardial infarction
2. Peripheral circulation and thermoregulation
   a. Abnormal vasomotor changes to:
      (i) vasoactive drugs
      (ii) temperature change
   b. Abnormalities of sweating
3. Gastrointestinal (Scarpello and Sladen 1978)
   a. Oesophagus – decreased strength of peristaltic contractions and decreased lower oesophageal sphincter tone (Hollis et al 1977)
   b. Stomach: delayed gastric emptying reduced incidence of peptic ulcer (Baron 1974) reduced gastric acid output Hosking et al 1975)
   c. Gallbladder atony (Grodzki et al 1968)
   d. Diarrhoea
4. Genitourinary system (Annals of Internal Medicine 1980)
   a. Loss of bladder sensation
   b. Impotence
   c. Failure of ejaculation
   d. Loss of testicular sensation (Campbell et al 1974)
5. Others
   a. Pupillary changes (Smith et al 1978)
   b. Cardiorespiratory arrest (Lancet Editorial 1978)
   c. Loss of awareness of hypoglycaemia

tion in perfusing the tissues of the limb. The autonomic nervous system also controls the rate of sweating and this is another important thermoregulatory mechanism. Changes in the autonomic control of both blood vessels and sweating can be demonstrated in diabetics.

A number of authors have demonstrated a reduced vasodilator response to body heating and reduced responses following the injection of vasoactive drugs. These changes were initially attributed to the presence of small vessel disease and the tests were advocated for its diagnosis, but a more likely explanation for the findings has been given by Moorhouse et al (1966) who studied the responses of the peripheral circulation to changes in temperature. They found that in subjects with chronic sympathetic denervation as occurs in diabetics, reflex responses which are related to requirements of internal temperature homeostasis did not occur. Instead, the vessels exhibited a local autonomy which was dependent on local temperature. Thus, vessels which did not dilate in response to heating the trunk would dilate if the limb were immersed in warm water. In addition the vasoconstriction which followed immersion of the foot in cold water was intense and prolonged.

Abnormalities in vasomotor function can be demonstrated by other stimuli. The wide local vasodilation or flare which is part of the triple response to injury depends on a local nervous reflex and may be absent in diabetics. The possible implications of this change are discussed in Chapter 5. A sudden deep breath will cause peripheral vasoconstriction by a reflex which passes through the thoracic spinal cord. The response to this test is also reduced in diabetics. The sudden application of ice to the face or neck will cause peripheral vasoconstriction

(Jamieson et al 1971), and a reduced response can be demonstrated in the lower limbs of diabetics with neuropathy.

The production of sweat can also be abnormal. It may be studied by heating the patient and coating the area to be examined with a material, such as quinizarin or starch-iodine powder, which changes colour when in contact with sweat. Various patterns of abnormal sweating in diabetic subjects have been described (Odel et al 1955). These may affect the trunk and head and neck, as well as the limbs, and have a patchy distribution. A further method for study is to measure the resistance to a small current passed through the skin. This is called the galvanic skin response and is a useful index of sympathetic nervous activity. Areas of abnormal resistance have been demonstrated in patients with diabetes and, as expected, these changes tend to parallel the changes of somatic neuropathy. Hyperhydrosis of the upper part of the body may be compensatory following loss of the ability of the lower limbs to sweat. Abnormal sweating of the face which follows eating (Watkins 1973) is probably due to local nerve abnormality (auriculotemporal nerve) rather than necessarily being part of a widespread change.

A selection from the tests described may be used if the aim is to study peripheral autonomic function. In recent years much interest has been focussed on detecting autonomic denervation of the heart. This has important clinical implications because of the incidence of painless myocardial infarction and of cardiorespiratory arrest in diabetic patients. There are now a battery of simple tests available (for details see Clarke et al 1979) which are dependent on the detection of heart rate and blood pressure changes in response to a variety of cardiovascular stimuli.

Beat-to-beat variation in heart rate
The variation which occurs in heart rate in normal subjects is largely due to changes in vagal activity in response to afferent stimuli from pulmonary stretch receptors. This variation is reduced in autonomic neuropathy. It can be assessed in several ways. (a) Maximal variation in heart rate can be induced by deep breathing at the rate of 6 breaths per minute. In normal subjects the rate varies by 15 or more beats per minute under this stimulus (Fig. 4.1). This is probably the test of choice (Mackay et al 1980). (b) The shorter stimulus of a single maximal inspiration followed by exhalation will produce a transient fall in heart rate. The change will be less in a patient with a denervated heart. (c) The standard deviation of the heart rate may be measured over a specified period, e.g. 5 minutes. In this case the standard deviation will be large in the normal subjects and small in those whose heart rate varies least.

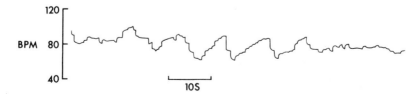

Fig. 4.1 Heart rate changes during deep breathing. Normal subject. There is an accentuation of the normal sinus arrythmia

Valsalva manoeuvre

This is the classic manoeuvre for studying autonomic reflexes affecting the circulation. Complete evaluation of the response requires arterial pressure monitoring (Fig. 4.2) but the heart rate changes provide a reliable guide to the circulatory changes. The patient maintains an expiratory pressure of 30 mm mercury for 10–15 seconds. In normal subjects the heart rate increases during this period. Following relaxation, the heart rate continues to rise for a few beats and then a profound bradycardia develops. It is the reduction or absence of this bradycardia which is the characteristic finding in autonomic neuropathy (Fig. 4.3). This test has the advantages of being simple, non-invasive and reproducible, and is within the capacity even of frail subjects.

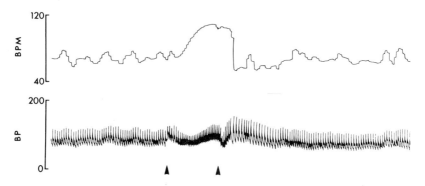

Fig. 4.2 Valsalva manoeuvre. Blood pressure and heart rate changes in a normal subject. There are several phases of the response

1. An initial rise in blood pressure as the rise in intrathoracic pressure is transmitted to the great vessels (first arrow).

2. A fall in blood pressure due to reduced venous filling of the heart. This results in a baroreflex-induced tachycardia with restoration of blood pressure.

3. When the pressure is released (second arrow) there is a sudden increase in filling of the heart. Cardiac output rises and so does the blood pressure ('overshoot'). This produces a bradycardia mediated via the baroreflexes.

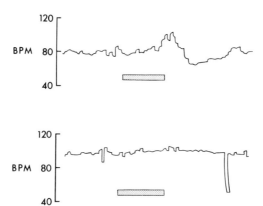

Fig. 4.3 Valsalva manoeuvre. Heart rate changes in a normal subject (above) and in a diabetic (below). In the diabetic the only change is a small increase in heart rate during the 10s period of the stimulus (indicated by the shaded marker). Note the higher resting heart rate in the diabetic.

Postural changes in blood pressure and heart rate

When one stands from a lying position there is pooling of blood in the legs which produces a fall in venous return and thus cardiac output. The normal compensatory responses are tachycardia and peripheral vasoconstriction both of which tend to maintain the normal blood pressure. In autonomic neuropathy there is a smaller rise in heart rate and, in addition, because there is reduced peripheral vasoconstriction, the blood pressure falls. Both the heart rate and blood pressure changes are easy to detect without arterial cannulation. An abnormal blood pressure response results in a fall of greater than 30 mm mercury.

Blood pressure response to isometric exercise

During isometric exercise the blood pressure and heart rate rise. The afferent stimuli arise from exercising muscles and the effector mechanisms involve a reduction in vagal tone on the heart and peripheral vasoconstriction. In response to a standard exercise (e.g. sustaining 30% of maximum voluntary contraction), a rise in diastolic blood pressure of less than 10 mm mercury is considered to be abnormal.

Table 4.2 summarizes the results of these tests.

Dyrberg et al (1981) have demonstrated using these tests, that autonomic neuropathy was present in 27% of 75 male, insulin-dependent diabetics (mean age 40, duration of diabetes 0–40 years). Neuropathy increased in frequency with the duration of the disease and was more prevalent in patients with nephropathy and proliferative retinopathy.

Table 4.2 Bedside tests of autonomic function

	Normal	Borderline	Abnormal
Beat-to-beat changes Max-min rate b p m	>15	11–14	<10
Standard deviation of the R R interval m s	>50		
Valsalva ratio	>1.20	1.11–1.20	<1.10
Postural change HR b p m	>1.03	1.01–1.03	<1.00
BP Fall in diastolic BP mmHg	<10	11–29	>30
Isometric exercise Rise in diastolic BP mmHg	>15	10–15	<10

EFFECTS ON THE FOOT

The foot is affected by damage to each of the types of fibres in the peripheral nerves.

Sensory changes

The changes described above range from lack of perception of vibration on the toes and at the ankles, to severe degrees of inability to feel painful stimuli. Once impairment of perception of pain has occurred, the foot is vulnerable to injury.

The mechanisms include burns from hot water bottles, injuries from foreign materials, e.g. pins in shoes, pressure from ill-fitting shoes and even pressure from adjacent toes. The common feature in all these examples is a failure to perceive the presence of a harmful agent which, in a normal patient, would be noticed by the pain it caused and therefore be removed. Have you ever tried to walk with a stone in your shoe? In the most severe cases spreading infection, large ulcers and even atherosclerotic gangrene are tolerated by the patient either with symptoms of a mild ache in the foot or without any complaint of pain.

Motor changes

Denervation of muscles has important effects on the function of the foot. The small muscles of the foot, the extensor digitorum brevis, lumbrical and interosseus muscles are commonly affected. The actions of these muscles are similar to those of the corresponding muscles in the hand. Their main function is to modulate the function of the long flexor and extensor muscles whose muscle bellies are remote from the site at which their tendons insert. The results of paralysis of the small muscle in the foot are analogous to the changes produced by denervation of the small muscles of the hand, e.g. by division of the deep branch of the ulnar nerve. The metatarsophalangeal joints are hyperextended and the interphalangeal joints are flexed. The joints initially remain mobile but later degenerative changes occur and the joints become fixed.

The deformity produced by the denervation which occurs predisposes to the development of ulcers. As the toes become clawed abnormal pressure may develop on the tips and occasionally ulcers form there. More often trauma occurs to the dorsum of the flexed and dorsally displaced proximal interphalangeal joint. A similar deformity may occur in non-diabetics. It probably results from muscle weakness associated with ageing but, apart from callus formation over the flexed interphalangeal joint, seldom causes any serious difficulties for the patient. The reason for the difference between diabetic and non-diabetic is that the former have pain sensation in the area and thus small injuries are noticed and treated. In the diabetic with neuropathy progressive tissue damage may occur.

Autonomic changes

The autonomic nerves provide vasoconstrictor and sudomotor fibres to the skin of the foot. The ways in which autonomic dysfunction can be demonstrated have been described above (see p. 31). There are a number of ways in which autonomic neuropathy might make the foot more vulnerable to injury or infection. It should be pointed out that these mechanisms are speculative rather than being established as important factors. They include (a) Failure of vasodilatation as part of the local response to injury which may predispose to the establishment of infection. (b) Abnormalities in the response to temperature changes (p. 30) which might be important if, for example, prolonged vasoconstriction in response to cold produced local hypoxia and the growth of anaerobic bacteria were favoured. (c) Loss of sweating which might produce changes in the pH and chemical environment of the skin and this might impair the skin defences against infection and alter the resident bacterial flora of the skin.

Trophic changes

This term is used to describe changes in the skin which result from denervation. A number of features are commonly described under this heading including redness and shininess of the skin and loss of hair (which is related neither to arterial disease nor to neuropathy). None of these are useful or important physical signs. However signs of increased pressure or friction are important because they represent the earliest stages of lesions which may develop into ulcers. The increased pressure which follows the altered mechanics of the foot causes areas of increased load to form under the areas of the metatarsal heads. Usually one area is predominantly involved. This increased load causes atrophy of the underlying subcutaneous tissue so that the metatarsal heads are relatively prominent. The skin becomes very thickly keratinised, often to a thickness of 5 mm or more. Breakdown of the skin in these areas produce ulcers (see p. 65).

Changes in joints

In patients with denervated joints, a non-infective joint degeneration which results in disorganization of the joint may occur. These changes were first described by Charcot in 1868 in a patient with locomotor ataxia (tabes dorsalis). They have since been described in many conditions in which there is loss of sensory innervation of a joint. They are commonly called Charcot or neuropathic joints regardless of the cause. Joints of the lower limb are predominantly affected. Those usually involved are the metatarsophalangeal joints and the joints between the tarsal and metatarsal bones. Occasionally the ankle and knee joints are affected and there are reports of involvement of the upper limb and spine. This degeneration may occur over a period of weeks or months during which the patient may complain of redness, swelling and occasionally pain in the affected area. For these changes to occur there must be sufficient blood supply to allow the hyperaemia. There is no established treatment which will halt this degeneration although a period of rigid immobilization might slow its progression. The hyperaemia subsides and the final result is a painless deformity.

The radiological appearances vary with the area involved. The features seen in a typical case include both destructive and hypertrophic changes. There is loss of joint space, and fragmentation and absorption of subchondral bone. Large osteophytes form at the joint margins and these may fracture. The appearances are of severe disorganization of the joint. In the diabetic the tarsal bones are most often affected by this process and the resulting appearances may suggest that one of the bones, e.g. the navicular, has almost completely disappeared. The appearances are different when the distal parts of the metatarsal bones or the phalanges are affected and these changes are sometimes described as 'atrophic'. There is destruction of the epiphyseal bone of the metatarsal heads and phalanges (Fig. 4.4). The shafts of the bones may be thinned with the result that the metatarsal shaft tapers to a pointed end. These changes may be difficult to distinguish from those associated with infection but if there is an ulcer beneath an affected joint infection of the joint should be assumed. In addition, if there is clinical evidence of infection in the foot, the joint is likely to be involved. Healing of the foot may occur in the absence of acute infection but should healing not occur, gen-

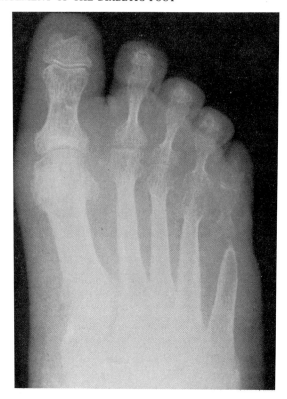

Fig. 4.4 Radiograph showing neuropathic, destructive changes of the fifth metatarsal head. Note partial destruction of distal phalanyx of great toe.

tle probing of the ulcer will usually reveal a communication with the underlying bone. In these circumstances the infected bone should be excised (see Ch. 10).

The importance of these changes in a diabetic is that any deformity of the foot may mean that parts are exposed to abnormally high pressure and friction forces. Because of the neuropathy these abnormal stresses are not perceived and very often ulcers occur over the affected joint. The management of these feet places a great strain on the resources of both chiropodist and bootmaker. Once ulcers occur, spontaneous healing is unlikely and recurrent ulceration frequently follows short periods of healing.

REFERENCES

Annals of Internal Medicine 1980 92 (Part 2): 291–342
Baron J H 1974 Letter: Autonomic neuropathy and autovagotomy. British Medical Journal 3: 408–409
Behse F, Buchtal F, Carlsen F 1977 Nerve biopsy and conduction studies in diabetic neuropathy. Journal of Neurology Neurosurgery and Psychiatry 40: 1072–1082
Bennett T, Hosking D J, Hampton J R 1980 Cardiovascular responses to graded reductions of central blood volume in normal subjects and in patients with diabetes mellitus. Clinical Science 58: 193–200
Campbell I W, Ewing D J, Clarke B F, Duncan L J P 1974 Testicular pain sensation in diabetic autonomic neuropathy. British Medical Journal 2: 638–639

Clarke B F, Ewing D J, Campbell I W 1979 Diabetic autonomic neuropathy. Diabetologia 17: 195–212

Clements R S 1979 Diabetic neuropathy – new concepts of its etiology. Diabetes 28: 604–611

Colby A O 1965 Neurologic disorders of diabetes mellitus. Diabetes 14: 424–429

Duchen L W, Anjorin A, Watkins P J, Mackay J D 1980 Pathology of autonomic neuropathy in diabetes mellitus. Annals of Internal Medicine 92 (Part 2): 301–303

Dyrberg T, Benn J, Christiansen J S, Hilsted J, Nerup J 1981 Prevalence of diabetic autonomic neuropathy measured by simple bedside tests. Diabetologia 20: 190–194

Editorial, Lancet: Cardiac death in diabetes. Lancet 1978 1: 1241–1242

Ewing D J, Campbell I W, Clarke B F 1976 Mortality in diabetic autonomic neuropathy. Lancet 1: 601–603

Fagerberg S–E 1959 Diabetic Neuropathy. Acta Medica Scandinavia Suppl 345: 1–80

Fraser D M, Campbell I W, Ewing D J, Murray A, Neilson J M M, Clarke B F 1977 Peripheral and autonomic nerve function in newly diagnosed diabetes mellitus. Diabetes 26: 546–550

Fraser D M, Campbell I W, Ewing D J, Clarke B F 1979 Mononeuropathy in diabetes mellitus. Diabetes 28: 96–101

Grodzki M, Mazurkiewicz-Rozynska E, Czyzyk A 1968 Diabetic cholecystopathy. Diabetologia 4: 345–348

Harrison M J G, Faris I B 1976 The neuropathic factor in the aetiology of diabetic foot ulcers. Journal of the Neurological Sciences 28: 217–223

Hollis J B, Castell D O, Braddom R L 1977 Esophageal function in diabetes mellitus and its relation to peripheral neuropathy. Gastroenterology 73: 1098–1102

Hosking D J, Moody F, Stewart I M, Atkinson M 1975 Vagal impairment of gastric secretion in diabetic autonomic neuropathy. British Medical Journal 2: 588–590

Jakobsen J 1978 Peripheral nerves in early experimental diabetes. Diabetologia 14: 113–119

Jamieson G G, Ludbrook J, Wilson A 1971 The response of hand blood flow to distant ice application. The Australian Journal of Experimental Biology and Medical Science 49: 145–152

Jordan W R 1936 Neuritic manifestations in diabetes mellitus. Archives of Internal Medicine 57: 307–366

Low P A, Walsh J C, Huang C Y, McLeod J G 1975 The sympathetic nervous system in diabetic neuropathy. Brain 98: 341–356

Mackay J D, Page M McB, Cambridge J, Watkins P G 1980 Diabetic autonomic neuropathy: the diagnostic value of heart rate monitoring. Diabetologia 18: 471–478

Mayne N 1965 Neuropathy in the diabetic and non-diabetic populations. Lancet 2: 1313–1316

Moorhouse J A, Carter S A, Douie J 1966 Vascular responses in diabetic peripheral neuropathy. British Medical Journal 1: 883–888

Odel H M, Roth G M, Keating F R 1955 Autonomic neuropathy simulating the effects of sympathectomy as a complication of diabetes mellitus. Diabetes 4: 92–98

Raff M C, Salgalang V, Asbury A K 1968 Ischemic mononeuropathy multiplex associated with diabetes mellitus. Archives of Neurology (Chicago) 18: 487–499

Scarpello J H B, Sladen G E 1978 Progress report: diabetes and the gut. Gut 19: 1153–1162

Smith S E, Smith S A, Brown P M, Fox C, Sönksen P H 1978 Pupillary signs in diabetic autonomic neuropathy. British Medical Journal 2: 924–927

Thomas P K, Lascelles R G 1966 The pathology of diabetic neuropathy. Quarterly Journal of Medicine 35: 489–509

Thomas P K, Eliasson S G 1975 Diabetic neuropathy in peripheral neuropathy. Volume 2, Dyck P J, Thomas P K, Lambert E H (eds) W B Saunders, Philadelphia pp 956–981

Watkins P J 1973 Facial sweating after food: a new sign of diabetic autonomic neuropathy. British Medical Journal 1: 583–587

5

Infection and wound healing

These two topics are linked because the ability to mount an inflammatory response is an essential component of both the wound healing process and the mechanisms of resistance to infection. In addition, wound infection is an important cause of failure of wound healing. The increased liability for diabetics to develop infections became part of the conventional wisdom in much the same way as the susceptibility to vascular disease. As with vascular disease, so have the beliefs about infection been challenged. Several large series have demonstrated that diabetes is a risk factor for the development of wound infection following operation (Cruse and Foord 1973). However Howard (1964) concluded that when allowance was made for the age of the subjects, the increased risk attributable to diabetes was no longer present. In addition many diabetics are obese and this, too, predisposes to the development of wound infection. The statistical techniques used in the reported studies have not been adequate to show if diabetes was a primary risk factor independent of, for example, age and obesity. Whatever the true situation, the important practical point is that the risk of infection is not so high as to preclude the safe performance of elective surgical procedures on patients with diabetes.

Infection is an important contributing factor to the morbidity of diabetic patients with foot problems. It is uncertain if they have a greater susceptibility to infection as a result of impaired resistance, or whether reduced blood supply allows infections to become established and the neuropathy permits the infection to go unrecognized. In any case the feet are now the commonest site for infection in diabetics and there is an excess representation of diabetics in groups of patients with deep infections of the foot.

Other forms of infection are also reported to be more common in diabetics. These groups include staphylococcal skin infections (particularly carbuncles), osteomyelitis, non-specific renal infections and renal tuberculosis, and certain fungal infections, e.g. vulval candidiasis. Infection was, in the pre-antibiotic era, a particularly feared complication of amputation in diabetics and the desire to be free of infected tissue was one of the reasons why high amputations were regularly performed in these patients.

MECHANISMS

The events which begin with an injury and end with the repair of the damage are a continuous sequence in which each successive change is dependent on the satisfactory progress of the preceding changes. However it is convenient to separate the process into artificially separate sections. Diabetes might lead to the impairment of the inflammatory and wound healing processes by reducing:

a. the blood supply to the affected area
b. the effectiveness of the inflammatory response
c. the repair process which results in the formation of fibrous tissue.

Impairment of blood supply

The pathological changes which occur in blood vessels in diabetes are described in Chapter 3. In atherosclerosis failure of wound healing is one of the characteristic results of minor injuries. A reduced blood supply may be sufficient to maintain the viability of tissues protected by an intact skin, but it may not be able to increase sufficiently to permit healing of even small wounds and, as a result, necrosis and infection may follow. The detection of hyperaemia around an ulcer or wound is the basis of one of the special tests used to predict healing of ulcers on the leg and foot (see p. 94). Diabetics who develop severe atherosclerosis are prone to suffer from failure to heal wounds of the leg and foot in the same way as non-diabetics. In ischaemic tissue the growth of anaerobic organisms is favoured, particularly if there is concomitant growth of aerobes. The risk of gas gangrene following amputation in non-diabetics is well known, but in addition diabetics may develop a spreading myositis produced by non-clostridial anaerobes (see p. 43). This latter infection is only marginally less lethal than the former.

There are several mechanisms by which the microvascular changes in diabetes could impair the response to injury. Blockage of small blood vessels might prevent the blood flow from increasing sufficiently to allow healing. In addition the capillary basement membrane thickening might alter the permeability and thus interfere with leucocyte migration and fluid exudation. The microvascular disease seen on histological examination is patchy in its distribution and it is considered unlikely that ischaemia due to these changes is a major cause of impaired healing. The possible effects of capillary basement membrane thickening are considered in the next section.

The effects of denervation of the blood vessels might be more important. The initial vascular response to a skin injury is the 'triple-response' which consists of: (1) an initial capillary vasodilation in the affected area; (2) dilation of the arterioles in a wide surrounding area ('flare'). This phase is mediated via a local axon reflex; and (3) a weal due to increased permeability of local blood vessels. The development of the flare is abolished following sympathectomy and is reduced in subjects with diabetic autonomic neuropathy. In addition the response of the denervated vessels to other stimuli may also be abnormal: there is evidence of increased vasoconstriction in response to both catecholamines (denervation hypersensitivity) and cold (see p. 30), and these might provide significant obstacles for the local autoregulatory mechanisms to overcome. These responses may aid the development of infection because there is experimental evidence that local vasoconstriction produced, for example, by injection of adrenaline enhances the infectivity of bacteria.

Formation of fluid-cellular exudate

The next phase of the inflammatory response is the accumulation at the site of injury of both leucocytes, whose function is to ingest and destroy bacteria, and protein rich fluid which aids this task. This process can be broken down into a number of stages including transport to the site of inflammation, migration through vessel walls, recognition of the object of phagocytosis, ingestion, killing of bacteria and subsequent digestion of phagocytosed material (Fig. 5.1). The effectiveness of these measures depends not only on the intrinsic activities of the cells but also on complex groups of proteins in the blood which facilitate the processes.
There is evidence that several of these stages are impaired in diabetics.

1. Decreased adhesion of polymorphs to vessel walls and reduced rate of escape from vessels have been described. It is uncertain whether the defect is in the leucocytes or in the vessel wall. Earlier studies suggested that the level of the blood glucose did not influence these processes. However using an *in vitro* system Bagdade et al (1978) found that the adherence of granulocytes was decreased in hyperglycaemic patients. The abnormality was directly related to the level of fasting blood glucose and returned towards normal with treatment. More recently the same group (Bagdade and Walters 1980) have demonstrated the same effect in patients with milder hyperglycaemia treated with an oral hypoglycaemic agent.

2. The mobility of white cells towards a chemical stimulus (chemotaxis) is impaired (Mowat and Baum 1971). This change, which was not seen in all subjects, might have been genetically determined because it was present in the first degree relatives of patients with diabetes. In addition, abnormalities of chemotaxis could not be demonstrated in cells taken from normal subjects and placed in hyperglycaemic medium, although the defect in the cells could be reversed by incubating with insulin.

3. The ability of the polymorphs to ingest and kill bacteria is reduced. (For review see Robertson and Polk, 1974). The first step in these processes is the recognition of the foreign material. This is facilitated by the activity of antibodies or

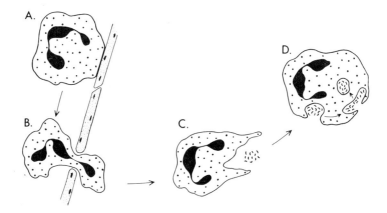

Fig. 5.1 Stages in the cellular response to inflammation.
  A. Adhesion to capillary wall
  B. Migration through wall
  C. Progression towards bacteria (Chemotaxis)
  D. Ingestion and destruction of bacteria (Phagocytosis)

other humoral factors, e.g. the complement system. The phagocytic cell then sends out pseudopodia to envelop the organism which comes to lie in a vacuole within the cell. The granules in the cell which contain various enzymes for the killing of bacteria and the digestion of foreign material then enter the vacuole. These changes are accompanied by a burst of oxidative activity within the cell. This results in the production of unstable compounds which produce oxidization of material within the vacuoles.

Although the various reports are not unanimous in their conclusions, it is likely that the leucocytes from hyperglycaemic patients are less efficient at both engulfing and killing bacteria. This defect may be improved by more rigorous control of the diabetes (Nolan et al 1978). It is probable that this inefficiency is at least in part due to impairment of energy production at the stage when normal cells show a burst of oxidative metabolism.

A very important component of the cellular response is the appearance of mononuclear cells which also have important phagocytic functions. Leibovich and Ross (1975) have demonstrated that impairment of monocyte function seriously impairs fibroblastic activity in experimental animals. Kitahara et al (1980) have demonstrated abnormal metabolic activity in monocytes from diabetics although it is not known if their *in vivo* activity is impaired.

The effect of ketosis has been studied by several groups with conflicting results. Some found that ketoacidosis was necessary before abnormalities of leucocyte function could be detected but other workers have demonstrated abnormalities in the absence of ketosis.

Formation of fibrous tissue

The changes of the inflammatory response described in the preceding sections are an essential preliminary to the formation of collagenous fibrous tissue. There is very little clinical evidence that wound healing, in the absence of infection, is less efficient in diabetics. A number of studies have shown differences between diabetics and non-diabetics in the rate of healing of foot amputations, but in these circumstances the adequacy of the blood supply is of critical importance and the published series do not always provide the data to assess this point.

In animal experiments the conditions are easier to control and Goodson and Hunt (1979) have reviewed the evidence which suggests that wound healing is impaired in insulin deficient animals.

The very earliest changes were examined by Arquilla et al (1976). They found a lack of DNA production close to the wound, reduced new capillary formation and decreased collagen production. These abnormalities were seen within four hours of wounding and emphasize the importance of the inflammatory response, abnormalities of which have been described in the previous sections. In longer term studies Goodson and Hunt (1979) demonstrated that the development of strength in an incised wound, which was closely related to the amount of collagen produced in the tissues closest to the wound edge, was decreased in insulin deficiency.

Insulin has been one of the many agents which are alleged to increase the rate of wound healing when applied topically in patients. However these types of studies face formidable difficulties in both their design and the assessment of the result. The experimental evidence is against its use in this way. Insulin did not increase the healing of granulating wounds (Rosenthal and Enquist 1968) and in tissue culture experiments the rate of collagen synthesis was dependent on the availability of glucose not insulin.

Thus there is good evidence that wound healing is impaired in the insulin deficient animal, although the evidence suggests that insulin lack does not directly influence the rate of collagen formation. It is likely that the effects of insulin deficiency on wound healing are due to the changes which occur in the earliest stages after wounding. The experiments of Goodson and Hunt demonstrated that granulation tissue formation could be returned to normal if insulin was given soon after wounding. If the insulin replacement was delayed until the time of greatest collagen formation (about 10 days after wounding) there was no increase in the amount of collagen formed. If this finding can be translated to humans it suggests that the greatest care should be taken to control the diabetes in the early postoperative period. In practice this is the time when good control is often most difficult to achieve. However in another model of diabetes, the obese mouse, Goodson and Hunt observed that insulin treatment of the hyperglycaemia did not restore collagen formation to normal. This has interesting implications for human subjects but great care is necessary in translating the results in these models to human disease.

This section has given details of a number of mechanisms by which resistance to infection and wound healing might be impaired and it is probable that both these defects are part of the syndrome of diabetes mellitus. However the effects of the abnormalities described are largely or totally reversible with treatment and in these circumstances the risks to the patient are not detectably greater than in a non-diabetic subject.

BACTERIOLOGY

The preceding account has discussed the host factors in the resistance to infection. Factors affecting the bacteria may also be important. *In vitro* high concentrations of glucose favour the multiplication of gram-positive bacteria, especially staphylococci, rather than gram-negative organisms. This matches the clinical observation (Robson 1970) that in patients with septicaemia gram-positive organisms were found in 80% of cases with a blood glucose level of greater than 7.2 mmol/l and gram-negative organisms in a similar proportion of patients with a lower blood glucose. It also supports the clinical observation that staphylococcal skin infections are more common in hyperglycaemic patients so that it is important to test for diabetes mellitus in any patient who presents with a carbuncle or repeated staphylococcal skin infections.

In the foot there are few specific features about the nature of the invading micro-organisms. The diabetic may suffer from the same sorts of infections which afflict non-diabetics. The common types include fungus infections of skin or nails. Fungus infections of the skin usually occur in moist areas of the foot and are often associated with poor hygiene. As such they should be regarded as a warning and an indication for encouragement and instruction to be given to the patient. The species most commonly involved are *tricophyton rubrum* and *interdigitale* and *epidermophyton flocculosum*. Paronychia may be fungal or staphylococcal and may be extensive if the foot is insensitive. Antifungal medication is adequate for the fungal type, but the staphylococcal infection will require drainage as well as antibiotic therapy.

The deep infections of the foot are the ones which are the most difficult to manage. There is nothing characteristic about the types of organisms found in the majority of cases. The commonest organisms have been described by Louie et al (1976) as including enterococci, staphylococci, clostridia and *escherichia coli*.

Spreading anaerobic infection is a very serious complication of a wound or an operation on the foot. The detailed clinical features are described on page 78 There are two groups of bacteria involved.

1. Clostridial

These are the same species which cause gas gangrene in non-diabetics — predominantly *clostridium perfringens* (Darke et al 1977) but in more than half the cases additional organisms can be cultured.

2. Non-clostridial

Non-clostridial anaerobic infections can occur in non-diabetics but are more common in diabetics. The organisms responsible include *e. coli*, bacteroides, anaerobic streptococci and all these organisms are commonly found contaminating lesions on the feet of diabetics. The infection should be differentiated from synergistic gangrene due to a combined infection with micro-aerophilic streptococci and *staphylococcus aureus*. This infection, which characteristically affects the perineum or abdominal wall, causes a spreading skin necrosis.

Therapy includes penicillin administration and amputation clear of the infected area. If hyperbaric oxygen therapy is available it may quickly limit the spread of the infection, the rapidity of the response being characteristic of clostridial infection. Further, if a rapid response is not obtained, the infection is unlikely to be clostridial and prolonging the hyperbaric therapy is unlikely to be of benefit (Darke et al 1977). This infection typically follows a major amputation for ischaemia. It is preventable by the preoperative administration of penicillin which should always be given to these patients. For the nonclostridial type it is important to recognize that antibiotic therapy is insufficient to prevent death and high amputation is required.

ANTIBIOTIC THERAPY

The major role for antibiotic therapy is to limit the spread of infection (see Table 5.1). This is important in two sets of circumstances.

    a. To limit the cellulitis which surrounds an abscess.

    b. To prevent the establishment of infection following surgery.

It will always be possible to grow bacteria from specimens obtained from open wounds. This is particularly true if, as in these patients, there is thick moist skin around the area or necrotic tissue in the base of the lesion. This does not mean that all patients must be given antibiotics. In most cases antibiotic therapy would be wasted because it is not possible to sterilize an area where dead tissue remains.

Table 5.1 Indications for antibiotic treatment

---

1. *Treatment of cellulitis*
   a. No abscess: curative
   b. Abscess present: limit spread of infection before drainage

2. *Prophylactic*
   a. Prior to local amputation: broad spectrum
   b. Prior to major amputation: penicillin

Equally antibiotic therapy is never sufficient treatment for an abscess because adequate drainage is always required. However, a knowledge of the flora in a particular patient is very important if appropriate antibiotic therapy is to be given and specimens should always be taken for culture in patients admitted to hospital for treatment of a foot ulcer, even though there may be no immediate indication for antibiotics. The detailed management of a patient with an abscess of the foot is discussed in Chapter 10. An important part of that management is the administration of antibiotics for 24–48 hours before operation. If a serious infection is present, antibiotic therapy will be required to combat a wide spectrum of organisms, and in most cases will be given before the results of cultures are available.

The choice of antibiotics for use depends on a knowledge of the types of organisms which may be present and on the clinical severity of the infection. Table 5.2 lists the antibiotics which may be administered and gives their usual doses. If a single agent is to be used, Cephoxitin is probably the best because of its activity against bacteroides species as well as the spectrum it shares with the other cephalosporins. Its disadvantage is a relative lack of activity against staphylococci. The combination of ampicillin and clindamycin may be used: ampicillin because of its activity against gram-negative organisms and clindamycin because of its effectiveness against enterococci, staphylococci and bacteroides. By comparison with clindamycin, lincomycin is less active against bacteroides but more active against clostridia. Penicillin is the agent of choice for the treatment of, or prophylaxis against, clostridial infection. Metronidazole has the great advantages of being nontoxic and active after administration either by mouth or by rectum.

Antibiotics used in this way are very effective at controlling the cellulitis. This has two important consequences for the patient. Firstly it minimizes the local tissue damage and secondly it reduces the size of the inflammatory focus so that the general condition of the patient improves and the diabetes becomes easier to control.

Table 5.2 Antibiotic therapy

---

1. *Treatment of an infected foot*
   Penicillin $1-2 \times 10^6$ units i.m. or i.v. 4–6 hourly
   Metronidazole 200 mg orally or rectally 8 hourly
   Ampicillin 500 mg orally or i.m. 6 hourly
   Clindamycin 300 mg orally or i.m. 6 hourly
   Cephoxitin 1–2 g i.v. 8 hourly
   Lincomycin 600 mg i.m. 6–12 hourly

2. *Prophylaxis of gas gangrene*
   Penicillin 1×10^6 units i.m. with premedication and 6 hourly for 24 hours
   In penicillin sensitive patients use Erythromycin 250 mg orally 6 hourly for 24 hours

---

The principle that antibiotic therapy, given preoperatively, will reduce the incidence of wound infections when the operation is carried out in a contaminated field is well established in surgical practice. Amputations performed close to an ulcer or area of gangrene in a diabetic patient are a very good illustration of the application of this principle. Freshly opened tissue planes are much more vulnerable than areas of granulation tissue to the establishment of infection. In order to be of benefit the antibiotics used must be effective against the likely types of potentially invasive bacteria. The cardinal principle, however, is that the blood must contain an adequate concentration of antibiotics at the time of operation. The question of timing is absolutely critical. Antibiotics which would reduce the chances of wound infection to very low levels if given preoperatively are much less effective if their administration is delayed for as little as 4 hours. This means that while antibiotics given 1 hour preoperatively are likely to be effective, it is often too late to give the same agents when the patient is in the recovery room after surgery. The other important practical point which has followed from these observations is that the duration of therapy, when used prophylactically, may be shorter than when established infection is being treated. Twelve-24 hours is all that is necessary in the former case while a 5-day course of therapy is commonly prescribed in the latter circumstances. However the circumstances in the wound following, for example, a ray amputation (see p. 104) in a diabetic patient are different from those following, say, an elective colectomy for neoplasm of the colon. In the latter case there may have been a heavy contaminating dose of bacteria during the operation but this risk is decreased when the anastomosis is completed and the skin wound closed. In the open wound on the diabetic foot, however, bacteria may multiply on the dressings at the same time as the exposed tissues are vulnerable to infection before granulation tissue forms. Because the foot is vulnerable for a longer time the course of antibiotics is often continued for 4–5 days.

Another very important use for antibiotics is in the prophylaxis of gas gangrene. All patients having a major amputation should have penicillin therapy before, and for 24 hours after, operation. By this means this dreaded complication can be avoided.

REFERENCES

Arquilla E R, Weringer, E J, Nakajo M 1976 Wound healing: a model for the study of diabetic angiopathy. Diabetes 25: 811–819

Bagdade J D, Root R K, Bulger R J 1974 Impaired leukocyte function in patients with poorly controlled diabetes. Diabetes 23: 9–15

Bagdade J D, Stewart M, Walters E 1978 Impaired granulocyte adherence: a reversible defect in host defense in patients with poorly controlled diabetes. Diabetes 27: 677–681

Bagdade J D, Walters E 1980 Impaired granulocyte adherence in mildly diabetic patients: effects of tolazamide treatment. Diabetes 29: 309–311

Cruse P J E, Foord R 1973 A five-year prospective study of 23 649 surgical wounds. Archives of Surgery 107: 206–210

Darke S G, King A M, Slack W K 1977 Gas gangrene and related infection: classification, clinical features and aetiology, management and mortality. A report of 88 cases. British Journal of Surgery 64: 104–112

Goodson W H, Hunt T K 1979 Would healing and the diabetic patient. Surgery Gynecology and Obstetrics 149: 600–608

Howard J M 1964 Ad Hoc Committee. Postoperative wound infections: the influence of ultraviolet irradiation of the operating room and of various other factors. Annals of Surgery Vol 160 Suppl

Kitahara M, Eyre H J, Lynch R E, Rallison M L, Hill H R 1980 Metabolic activity of diabetic monocytes. Diabetes 29: 251–256

Leibovich S J, Ross R 1975 The role of the macrophage in wound repair. A study with hydrocortisone and antimacrophage serum. American Journal of Pathology 78: 71–100

Louie T J, Bartlett J G, Tally F P, Gorbach S L 1976 Aerobic and anaerobic bacteria in diabetic foot ulcers. Annals of Internal Medicine 85: 461–463

Mowat A G, Baum J 1971 Chemotaxis of polymorphonuclear leukocytes from patients with diabetes mellitus. New England Journal of Medicine 284: 621–627

Nolan C M, Beaty H N, Bagdade J D 1978 Further characterization of the impaired bactericidal function of granulocytes in patients with poorly controlled diabetes. Diabetes 27: 889–894

Robertson H D, Polk H C Jr 1974 The mechanism of infection in patients with diabetes mellitus: a review of leukocyte malfunction. Surgery 75: 123–128

Robson M C 1970 A new look at diabetes mellitus and infection. American Journal of Surgery 120: 681–682

Rosenthal D P, Enquist I F 1968 The effect of insulin on granulating wounds in normal animals. Surgery 64: 1096–1098

6

Mechanical factors

The important role of physical factors in the development of ulcers has been mentioned in Chapter 2. The agents involved are largely mechanical although thermal and chemical factors may occasionally be important. The effect of all these agents is aided by, and may depend on, loss of perception of pain in the foot. The mechanical forces (Fig. 6.1) may act by:
   a. Disrupting tissue
   b. Pressure causing ischaemia
   c. Repetitive stress causing necrosis

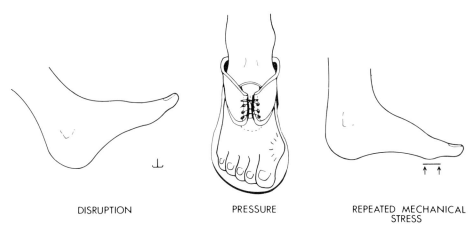

DISRUPTION   PRESSURE   REPEATED MECHANICAL
                                                                STRESS

Fig. 6.1 Mechanical causes of foot lesions

Disruption
Localized high pressure may cause disruption of tissue — a large force is required and this must be applied to a small area. Treading on broken glass or a drawing pin are examples of this sort of force. The best way that a patient can protect himself is to always wear footwear so that the chances of these accidents is much reduced.

Ischaemic necrosis from pressure
When one stands, the pressure between some parts of the foot and the surface will be sufficient to stop the blood supply to those areas. Another example of this phenomenon is seen in contracting muscle, e.g. the heart, when the tension de-

veloped during contraction stops perfusion. This is normal and quite harmless. However, if moderate pressure is applied to an area of skin for a prolonged period, ischaemic necrosis of this area may result. One common example is the formation of a bedsore.

This is an important mechanism for the development of lesions in diabetic patients. The forces required are not high, 1–2 lb f/in^2 (7–14kPa) is sufficient (Brand 1978), but it must be maintained for several hours. If the arterial supply is reduced, the pressure required to stop the skin circulation will be less, thus atherosclerosis is an additional predisposing factor. There are two situations in which ischaemic necrosis commonly occurs in diabetics. The first is trauma from wearing a new pair of shoes (see Fig. 8.3). The lesions occur at the sides of the foot, over the first metatarsal head, the interphalangeal joint of the great toe or the base of the fifth metatarsal bone. Because the duration of the pressure is critical in the production of necrosis, adequate preventative measures are obvious and simple: new shoes should never be worn for longer than two hours until they are well adjusted to the shape of the foot. At the end of this time the shoes and socks should be removed and the feet carefully inspected. Affected areas will be pale initially but the skin reddens as reactive hyperaemia develops. The appearance of such an area means that the particular pair of shoes should not be worn any longer that day. The second situation in which ischaemic necrosis occurs is on the pressure areas around the heel and malleoli in a patient who has decreased sensation in the feet and who is in bed for a prolonged period. Here both factors, namely low pressure and its prolonged application, are acting. The presence of occlusive arterial disease also potentiates the development of ischaemic necrosis in these patients. Prevention depends on diligent nursing which gives regular attention to pressure areas.

Repetitive stress
The idea that lesions might be produced by moderate repetitive stress with pressures which neither disrupt the tissues nor cause ischaemic necrosis has made much clearer our understanding of the development of the common neuropathic ulcer (Brand 1978). This concept provides a coherent explanation for the sequence of events which leads to the development of an ulcer. A detailed account of the factors involved is given because of its importance and because a unified account of the various factors cannot easily be found elsewhere. The following account is in two parts:
   1. the mechanics of walking and
   2. abnormalities in diabetes which lead to the formation of ulcers.

MECHANICS OF THE FOOT

With the assumption by man of the erect posture, the foot became subject to a variety of stresses which were not encountered by our arboreal ancestors. The evolutionary and adaptive processes are neither complete nor perfect, e.g. the lateral metatarsal bones may fracture with repeated minor trauma (stress fracture). The analysis of the functions of the lower limb during walking has proved difficult although a large number of techniques have been brought to bear including gross anatomical studies, electromyography, cine-radiology and cinematography, and engineering approaches to the study of load. It is the purpose of this section to consider the mechanical forces on the foot, the abnormalities which may occur in diabetics and the way which the stresses may be modified in the treatment of these patients.

The movements of the ankle and associated joints will only be mentioned briefly and more proximal joints not discussed at all in this account.

Anatomical factors

A casual glance at skin of the foot will immediately reveal one of the most important adaptations for weight bearing namely the production of keratin. The keratin is thickest on those parts of the foot which carry the greatest load and this is especially noticeable on the heel. Keratin production adapts very quickly to changed loads: it will increase during a seaside holiday if one walks barefoot and will decreases if the leg is immobilized in plaster so that on resumption of walking the skin is soft and tender. If an area of abnormal load develops, e.g. as a result of neuropathic change in an underlying joint, the response is for excess keratin to develop at that site. This is a normal response to increased load. There is no increased tendency for diabetics to produce keratin: it is the load which is abnormal not the response.

The subcutaneous tissue is dense with many fibrous bands between the lobules of fat. It is also very strong and resistant to acute trauma, e.g. a fall may result in a fracture of the calcaneum but the overlying skin appears undamaged. However repeated abnormal stress may result in atrophy of the subcutaneous tissue so that the underlying bones come to lie closer to the skin.

The bones ligaments and fasciae of the foot are obviously of fundamental importance in walking and their functional anatomy has been studied by many people. The longitudinal arches formed by the tarsal and metatarsal bones differ in several important ways from architectural arches. Firstly the arches of the foot are flexible and change their shape when under load. Secondly the stresses on the arches of the foot produce bending stresses on the plantar aspect whereas on a masonry arch there are purely compressive forces acting. This fact is easily confirmed anatomically by the relative thickness of the plantar as compared to the dorsal ligaments of the foot. The plantar aponeurosis has an important role in preventing excessive displacement of the pillars of the arches, viz. the calcaneum and the metatarsal heads. Much attention has been given to the so called windlass action of this fascia (see Fig. 6.2). The anterior attachments of the fascia are in the digits so that when the toes are dorsiflexed, as they are during walking just before the foot leaves the ground, there is increased tension in the fascia and this tends to approximate the pillars of the arch. Fixed shortening of this fascia, which may occur in diabetics as a result of dorsal displacement of the toes (see p. 55), may result in a permanently high-arched foot (pes cavus). This has the additional effect of increasing the loads carried by the area of the metatarsal heads. Studies of the load carried by the foot produce no support for the idea of a functionally important transverse arch at the level of the metatarsal heads: indeed it is often true that the middle metatarsals carry greater loads than the first and fifth bones. The actions of the muscles inserting in the foot may be different during walking

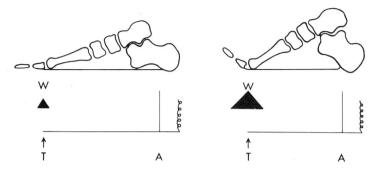

Fig. 6.2 Figure showing (left) how fixed dorsiflexion of the toes will result in shortening of the longitudinal arch through the attachments of the plantar fascia. (Right) If the distance TA is shortened a given force applied to the spring will result in a greater load at T (see p.55).

to those inferred from a study of their attachments in the cadaver. An account of some of these actions is given in the following section.

Gait

The investigation of the mechanics of walking includes two groups of observations. These are the study of the geometry of the changes which occur in the leg and foot, and the analysis of the forces exerted. Walking involves the co-ordinated action of many parts of the body, particularly of the whole of the lower limbs. This account is confined to a description of the actions directly affecting the foot.

A walking cycle is defined as the time between the heel making contact with the ground and the time immediately before the same heel makes contact with the ground the next time. Each foot is in contact with the ground for about 60% of the walking cycle. Thus both feet are in contact with the ground from 0–10% of the cycle and from 50–60% of the cycle. The time during which the foot is in contact with the ground can be divided into three parts (Fig. 6.3).

1. Heel strike. This begins when the heel strikes the ground and ends when the forefoot comes into contact with the surface.

2. Stance. This is the longest of the periods and lasts while both heel and forefoot are in contact with the surface. It includes the time when the body weight is transferred forwards and ends when the heel leaves the ground.

3. Step-off. During this last phase the body weight is propelled forwards. The forefoot carries its greatest loads during this phase which ends when the foot leaves the ground.

The major movements of the ankle joint and foot are initiated by muscles which arise in the calf. Figure 6.3 shows a simplified version of the events during walking. The position of the ankle joint and the electrical activity of the major muscle groups are shown. During the heel-strike phase there is plantar flexion of the ankle joint which returns to a neutral position when the forefoot reaches the ground. These movements of the ankle are under the influence of gravity and the anterior tibial muscles. While the foot is in contact with the ground there is progressive dorsiflexion of the ankle as the body-weight is transferred forwards. This process is initiated by the anterior tibial muscles then continued by gravity and resisted by the posterior tibial and intrinsic foot muscles. During the step-off

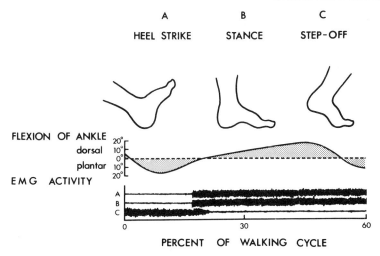

Fig. 6.3 The three phases of gait which occur while the foot is in contact with the ground. The lowest tracings illustrate the electrical activity in:
A. posterior calf muscles
B. intrinsic muscles of the foot
C. anterior calf muscles

phase there is progressive plantar flexion of the ankle until the foot is lifted from the ground. Denervation of the tibial muscles is seldom a problem in diabetics although in severe cases of neuropathy foot drop may occur due to lesions of the common peroneal nerve. More often the gait is ataxic because of sensory neuropathy which affects the joint position sense so that the precision with which the movements are performed is less. The intrinsic muscles of the foot, although not of great strength, have very important functions in modulating the action of the long flexor and extensor muscles. The extensor digitorum brevis and flexor digitorum accessorius muscle respectively influence the direction of action of the extensor digitorum longus and flexor digitorum longus muscles. As in the hand the lumbrical and interosseous muscles cause flexion of the metatarsophalangeal joint and extension of the interphalangeal joint (see p. 34). The intrinsic muscles have other functions which aid the maintenance of the integrity of the foot. They provide bulk and padding to cover the bones, they help maintain the arches, they provide the maximum surface area for the forefoot and they limit overextension of the metatarsophalangeal joints.

Forces under the foot

The forces between the foot and the shoe or ground with which it is in contact comprise both perpendicular or weight-bearing forces and horizontal and frictional forces. Much more is known about the weight bearing forces because they are much easier to measure than the frictional forces. The studies of weight bearing described below have provided information which helps to explain the distribution and occurrence of plantar ulceration. The following account is concerned with weight bearing forces.

The loads carried on the under surface of the foot will depend on the body weight and anatomical and functional properties of the foot such as the action of the muscles and the bony skeleton (and any abnormalities thereof).

The loads have been difficult to study precisely. Two types of methods have been used to obtain quantitative data. In the first, a load sensitive area is set into a walkway so that the forces exerted can be recorded during a single step or during stance. The objection to this method is that the loads recorded might not accurately reflect the forces acting between the foot and any footwear normally worn. This objection is overcome by placing transducers beneath the foot but inside the footwear. However this method has the limitations that only selected areas can be studied and, more importantly, the presence of transducers might affect the loads measured. Despite these limitations important information has been obtained using both techniques.

For a semi-quantitative study of relative loads the Harris mat is useful. This comprises a rubber mat with ridges at three different levels. The mat is inked and covered with paper on which the subject walks. The arrangement of the ridges is such that the densest impression is produced by the greatest load. This can be used either on the floor or a thin piece of the material can be placed inside the shoe. The latter method will give an idea of the load carried during walking in the patient's own shoe and this is likely to be a good guide to the stresses which the foot undergoes during daily activities. This technique has the great advantages of simplicity and ease of interpretation.

The most detailed information has been obtained from studies in which a force plate has been used. One such apparatus was described by Stokes et al (1974). This comprised 12 parallel beams each 11×400 mm from which simultaneous measurements of the load were made. The load on each beam represented the forces on a strip of the foot 11 mm wide during the step recorded. An inked pad was used to obtain a footprint which gave precise information about the part of foot in contact with each beam. By studying the course of events on a beam, the particular part of the foot in contact with the beam at any given time could be inferred. Figure 6.4 shows the loading pattern on the beams in one such study. Those beams with which the heel came in contact (5, 6, 7) recorded a rapid rise in load early in the cycle. This decreased as the load was transferred to the forefoot and rose again during the step-off phase when the heel left the ground and the metatarsal heads and toes were in contact with the beam. The peak load on the forefoot in this case was recorded earlier over the lateral side of the foot (beam 2) than on the medial side (beam 7), indicating that there had been a rolling movement of the foot from lateral to medial. The degree and direction of this movement varies between individuals. A histogram of the maximum loads on the forefoot (Fig. 6.5) shows that there was a reasonably even distribution of the load and in particular there were no areas of localized high load.

From the point of view of the loads carried, the foot may be arbitrarily divided into three areas: heel, mid-foot and forefoot. The forefoot includes the distal part of the metatarsals and the toes. The mid-foot includes the highest parts of the longitudinal arches. If the beams were arranged so that they were at right angles to the direction of walking the loads carried by heel, mid-foot, area of metatarsal heads and toes could be resolved. In normal subjects the load carried by the mid-foot was never greater than 10% of the body weight. This contradicts the conven-

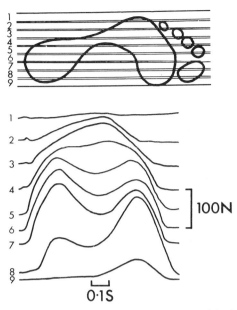

Fig. 6.4 Measurement of forces under the foot. (Above) The outline of the footprint shows which parts of the beams were in contact with the foot. (Below) Forces recorded from each beam. The left hand end of each line represents zero load

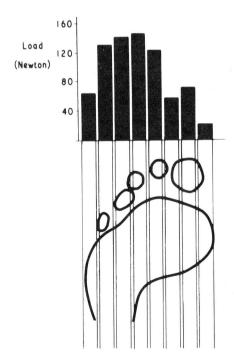

Fig. 6.5 Maximum forefoot loads. Normal foot. The highest loads are carried in the middle of the forefoot. There are no localized areas which carry high loads (cf. Figs. 6.7 and 6.8)

tional accounts which describe the transfer of the load as occurring along the lateral side of the foot. The toes normally carried about 30% of the body weight during the later stages of the step-off phase. More detailed information has been obtained following the recent development of a load sensitive area which contains 128 cells each 15 × 15 mm in area (Hutton and Dhanendran 1979). In normal subjects measurement of the maximum force has shown that the area of the 3rd–5th metatarsal heads carries a load equivalent to 35% of the body weight. The great toe, first and second metatarsal separately carry a maximum of 25% of the body weight. The second and third to fifth toes carry less than 10% of the body weight (Fig. 6.6)

Similar findings were reported by Bauman et al (1963) who attached transducers to five sites on the sole of the foot. These transducers were only 1 mm thick so that the distortion produced would be minimal. Their important contribution was to compare barefoot walking on various surfaces with walking using various types of footwear. They demonstrated that the loads measured from a particular area of the foot were less if the subject trod on leather than if the surface was concrete and least when on a rubber surface. Part of this difference may have been artefact

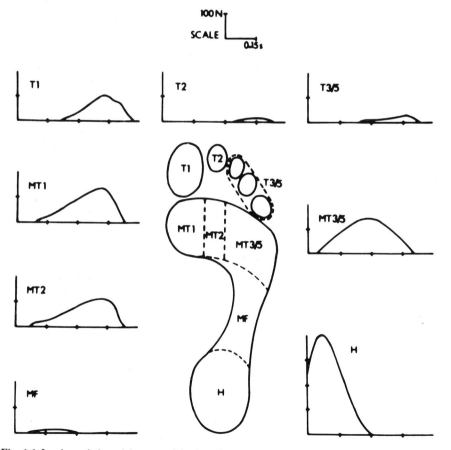

Fig. 6.6 Loads carried on eight areas of the foot during a single step. (Hutton and Dhanendran 1979)

due to the varying response of the transducer but there probably remained a real difference between the surfaces. They were also able to demonstrate differences in load carried by the areas of the foot when footwear of different patterns was worn. These findings will be discussed in more detail when the design of shoes is being considered (p. 67). The distribution of the body weight when standing has been the subject of conflicting accounts. Recent studies (Hutton et al 1976) demonstrated that there was a range of patterns, all compatible with comfortable stance, which might be adopted. The heel carried between one and three times the load carried on the forefoot, but the distribution of the load varied with the need to maintain balance.

CHANGES IN DIABETICS

The alterations which occur in diabetics in the loading of the foot are primarily the result of neuropathy although partial amputation of the foot may also produce effects equally as important. The effects of neuropathy have been discussed in detail in Chapter 4 (see p. 33). The important results are deformities produced by paralysis of the small muscles of the foot and by neuropathic degeneration of the joints. The former produces the claw-toe deformity and the latter may produce areas of high load in abnormal sites. They may have the important results of changing the distribution of forces under the foot. An understanding of these changes would not only help to explain the occurrence and distribution of foot ulcers, but also might direct attention to the sites which are at greatest risk for the development of ulcers.

The first effect of the clawing of the toes might be to shorten the base of the longitudinal arches of the foot by the windlass mechanism (see p. 49). This effective shortening of the foot would mean that contraction of the calf muscles would produce a greater force on the forefoot because of the shorter length involved (see Fig. 6.2). The pes cavus deformity is sometimes seen and this change in leverage may be important in these patients. However, more frequently there is no obvious pes cavus, presumably because the plantar fascia also gives way under the stress of the loads carried. The clawing also makes the toes more vulnerable to frictional forces.

Are areas of increased load detectable?   This has been studied by Stokes et al (1975) and there are several important conclusions to be drawn from this study. If an ulcer was present, the site of the ulcer always corresponded to the area of the forefoot which carried the highest load. In patients whose feet were deformed either by the presence of neuropathic joints or as a result of operation, e.g. ray amputation, abnormally high loads could be demonstrated over either the deformity (Fig. 6.7) or one or more prominent metatarsal heads (Fig. 6.8). In feet without ulcers, areas of abnormally high load could be demonstrated and these corresponded to the site of callus formation. In passing it should be noted that the maximum load was directly proportional to the body weight so that heavier patients may run greater risks of developing foot ulcers. The use of these measurements in the design of splints and prostheses is discussed on page 69. The sequence of events which occurs in diabetics and leads to foot ulcers can be reconstructed using this information. One or more areas of the forefoot, in the region of the meta-

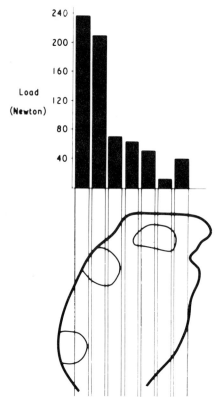

Fig.6.7 Abnormal loading pattern in a right foot which was deformed by neuropathic degeneration in the tarsal bones. There were ulcers present in both the areas represented by circles on the medial side of the foot.

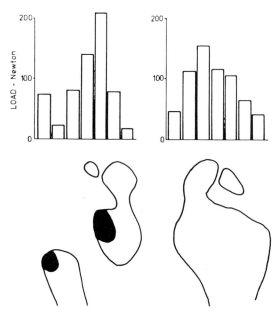

Fig. 6.8 Abnormal loading pattern in a patient following two ray amputations. Both the shaded areas which carried high loads subsequently became ulcers. The pattern in the right foot was normal.

tarsal heads or the interphalangeal joint of the great toe, come to carry greater than normal loads. This is an invariable precursor of the plantar ulcer. This increased load occurs for several reasons. First, the clawing of the toes means that they are unable to carry their normal load and thus the effective weight bearing surface of the forefoot is reduced in area. Second, paralysis and atrophy of the small muscles of the foot results in increased prominence of the metatarsal heads. Third, the lever effect due to shortening of the foot may be important in some cases.

The link between increased load and the development of ulcers has been given by Brand (1978) who demonstrated that moderate stresses applied repeatedly to hand or foot caused inflammation. The force needed was not large and those measured by Stokes et al (1975) were in the range which would produce these effects. In human subjects, Brand demonstrated that these stresses caused redness and tenderness which took more than 24 hours to resolve so that there was reduced tolerance of similar stresses the next day. Daily exposure to these forces in experimental animals produced continued inflammation and eventually necrosis and ulceration of the affected area.

A similar sequence is very likely in the feet of diabetics who for reasons given above, develop areas of local increase in the load carried. A foot which has normal sensation and which experiences these stresses is protected because the inflammation causes pain. As a result the subject relieves the stress either by resting or by altering the gait to reduce the load on the tender area. If the patient is unaware of this inflammation because of diabetic or other neuropathy, no action will be taken to relieve the load so that the stresses produced by walking continue, and progression to necrosis and ulceration may occur. The detection of these inflamed areas is an important step in the prevention of ulceration because, if adequate rest is given, resolution can occur. These areas can be seen as 'hot spots' on thermograms of the foot and their course followed by this method.

Fortunately changes in temperature can be detected by simpler techniques. Difference in skin temperature of 2°C can be detected normally (and this is in the range of temperature increase commonly found in these patients). It must be remembered that many patients have impairment of sensation in their hands as well as their feet. In these cases the feet should be palpated by another person who presumably has normal sensation. If more precision is required a thermistor is a sufficiently accurate method for measuring skin temperature.

REFERENCES

Bauman J H, Girling J P, Brand P W 1963 Plantar pressures and trophic ulceration. Journal of Bone and Joint Surgery 45B: 652–673
Brand P W 1978 Pathomechanics of diabetic (neurotrophic) ulcer and its conservative management. In Bergan J J and Yao J S T (eds) Gangrene and severe ischaemia of the lower extremities. Grune and Stratton, New York
Hutton W C, Stott J R R, Stokes I A F 1976 The mechanics of the foot. In Klenerman L (ed) The foot and its disorders. Blackwell, Oxford, pp 30–48
Hutton W C, Dhanendran M 1979 A study of the distribution of load under the normal foot during walking. International Orthopaedics 3: 153–157
Stokes I A F, Stott J R R, Hutton W C 1974 Force distributions under the foot — a dynamic measuring system. Biomedical Engineering 9: 140–143
Stokes I A F, Faris I, Hutton W C 1975 The neuropathic ulcer and loads on the foot in diabetic patients. Acta orthopaedica Scandinavica 46: 839–847

7

Prevention of major lesions

It is a major aim of the management of diabetics to prevent the development of complications of the disease amongst which foot lesions are an important source of morbidity. This aim too frequently fails and later chapters of the book will be concerned with the assessment and management of these failures. This chapter will consider the steps which may be taken to minimize the chances of development of a major lesion. The measures to be discussed include:

a. Routine care given to all diabetic patients

b. Details of the treatment of minor lesions and the non-operative treatment of ulcers

c. Provision of adequate footwear and the use of prostheses.

An account of the ways in which mechanical forces may affect the foot has been given in the preceding chapter, and the avoidance of these injuries is the prime topic of this section. This is, however, an appropriate time to consider the vexed question of the effect of control of the blood glucose concentration on the development of complications. Some of the arguments have been discussed in the chapters describing the individual complications of diabetes but a summary of the evidence is presented here.

ROUTINE CARE

Control of the diabetes

There is unanimous agreement that diabetes should be carefully controlled. However two major problems are immediately encountered. The first is to define and assess good control and the second is to demonstrate a resulting benefit. Perfect control of diabetes would be defined as maintaining the blood sugar at the same level as in a healthy person without diabetes. This aim will not be achievable until there are available insulin delivery systems which respond to the blood glucose levels. It is a matter of opinion as to how much deviation from the ideal state is allowable. Good control may be defined by setting acceptable levels of the blood glucose before and after meals but it must be remembered that blood sugar measurements taken at infrequent intervals do not indicate previous or subsequent fluctuations in concentration.

Great interest has been shown in the observation that glucose may become attached to the haemoglobin molecule to form a separately identifiable substance called haemoglobin A_{Ic} (HbA_{Ic}) (see p. 19). The process involves condensation of the glucose molecule with the N-terminal amino acids of the beta chain of the haemoglobin molecule. The rate of the reaction is a function of the blood glucose concentration. It occurs slowly (and is therefore reversed slowly) and continues for the life of the red cell. Thus the concentration of HbA_{Ic} in the blood might give some indication of the mean level of blood glucose over a period of weeks or months, related to the life of the red blood cell (see Koenig and Cerami 1980 for review). In contrast a single estimate of the blood glucose level provides only a brief glimpse of a rapidly changing scene. The exact importance of HbA_{Ic} estimations is still being determined. The account given above is too simple because there are wide differences between subjects in the rate of formation of HbA_{Ic} and the response to restoration of normoglycaemia (Brooks et al 1980).

The other major problem is that it has been difficult to produce strong evidence that careful regulation of the blood glucose influences the development of complications. There is much anecdotal evidence. Rapid progression of neuropathy may follow periods when the control of the diabetes has been recognized to be bad, and groups of patients in whom the diabetes has been rigorously controlled have been demonstrated to live for long periods without developing disabling microangiopathy (Chazan et al 1970).

The evidence supporting the view that good control reduces complications has been summarized by Tchobroutsky (1978).

Clinical studies
This is clearly the evidence on which the case will be made or broken. Most of the data presented has been criticized on statistical and epidemiological grounds and it must be conceded that this data certainly does not prove the hypothesis that good control prevents the development of complications. However, more recently the results of prospective studies have been reported and the balance of the conclusions from these studies is that good control slows the rate of deterioration of established lesions.

Experimental studies
There are a number of studies which have shown that the development of lesions associated with experimental diabetes may be slowed by insulin therapy and islet cell transplantation. However great care must be taken in extrapolating the results of these animal experiments to human disease.

Biochemical factors
Treatment of diabetes can be shown to reverse some of the biochemical or enzymatic changes which are part of the metabolic disturbance found in the disease. The difficulty is that although a plausible hypothesis for the development of complications can be created on the basis of these changes, there is no direct evidence establishing a casual relationship.

The difficulty of this problem can be seen by the controversy which followed the publication of a policy statement by the American Diabetic Association which concluded that 'the weight of the evidence, particularly that accumulated in the past five years, strongly supports the concept that the microvascular complications of diabetes are decreased by reduction of blood glucose concentration'

(Cahill et al 1976). This produced a vigorous response (Siperstein et al 1977) which concluded that 'we have yet to find clear evidence that insulin therapy, as currently applied, has altered the course of the microangiopathic lesions of diabetes'. The attempts to produce perfect control of the diabetes are not without risks. Hypoglycaemia is the most serious of these. It is the most frequent complication of long-standing diabetes and may have disastrous socio-economic effects on employment and, for example, the obtaining of a driver's licence. In addition it may cause short- and long-term neurological damage. There will also be additional costs to the patient and/or the community from the extra medical care needed to supervise the control of the diabetes, although these costs could be easily justified if the result was fewer complications of the disease.

How do the prudent clinician and patient act in the face of this uncertainty? There is general agreement that the diabetes should be controlled as carefully as possible without producing disabling hypoglycaemia. The vigour with which normoglycaemia is pursued will depend on the rapport between patient and advisors, the degree of insight shown by the patient, the brittleness of the diabetes, the need to avoid hypoglycaemia and finally the conclusion reached from a study of the evidence outlined above.

Care of the foot

Within 10 years of the discovery of insulin, special measures taken to care for the feet of diabetic patients were instituted, and it was demonstrated subsequently that the provision of a 'foot room' in a diabetic clinic had reduced the number of patients requiring admission to hospital, the number of amputations and the mortality (Brandaleone et al 1937). Care of the feet takes place at three levels:

   a. There are the routine measures which the patient must take to care for his feet.

   b. Early lesions require expert care either from a chiropodist or a doctor experienced in the care of these patients.

   c. Advanced lesions will require specialist surgical care.

The first two phases are the subject of this section. Detailed management of advanced lesions is given in chapter 10.

Role of the patient

The prevention of foot lesions requires the co-operation of the patient and it is likely that the better the patient is informed about the disease, the more he or she will be able to take a responsible part in the management. In this regard associations of diabetic patients have a very valuable role in providing a forum in which diabetics can learn from each other and through which information can be distributed.

Education of the patient is an essential function of all those caring for diabetics. Many clinics supply a list of printed instructions. An example of part of such a leaflet is shown in Figure 7.1. The guidance should be simple and straightforward and include information about the following aspects.

   1. General.   Diabetes may affect the nerves so that pain signals arising in the foot do not reach the brain. This means that the diabetic loses the warning signals produced by injury. The diabetic must therefore use the other senses, especially

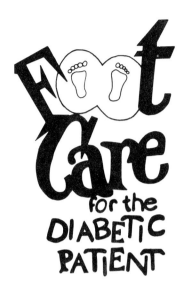

PROTECT
YOUR FEET BY . . . . .

AVOIDING EXPOSURE TO RAIN, COLD
AND EXCESSIVE SUNLIGHT

AND NEVER . . . . .

CUT CORNS AND CALLUSES WITH RAZOR-
BLADE OR KNIFE

APPLY A HOT WATER BOTTLE, A HEATING
PAD OR HOT WATER TO YOUR FEET

WEAR CUT OUT SHOES OR SANDALS

APPLY STRONG ANTISEPTIC OR CHEMICALS
TO YOUR FEET

DON'T BE FOOT FOOLISH !

IT IS ESSENTIAL THAT YOU KEEP YOUR
DIABETES UNDER GOOD CONTROL TO
ENSURE GOOD FOOT CARE

DISCUSS ALL FOOT PROBLEMS PROMPTLY
WITH YOUR PHYSICIAN OR PODIATRIST

Fig. 7.1 Part of the instruction leaflet issued by the Diabetic Clinic at the Royal Adelaide Hospital

the eyes and hands to detect the earliest signs of injury or infection because if these are neglected serious problems may develop.

2. Daily inspection.   Inspect the feet every day. Seek advice if any swelling, cracks in the skin, redness or sores are present.

3. Protection of feet.   Never walk barefooted. Avoid casual footwear or sandals which leave the toes exposed.

4. Shoes.   Leather shoes, although more expensive, are preferred because they more easily conform to the shape of the foot than shoes made from synthetic materials. They must not cause abnormal pressure on any part of the foot. Shoes which try to make the foot conform to the currently fashionable shape must be avoided.

A new pair of shoes should not be worn for longer than two hours on the first occasion. At the end of that time remove the shoes and inspect the feet for any signs of redness or warmth which indicate that the area has been exposed to abnormal pressure or friction.

Develop the habit of inspecting and feeling the inside of each shoe for nails or foreign material before putting it on.

No pair of shoes should be worn for longer than 4 or 5 hours if this can be avoided.

5. Socks.   Woollen or heavy cotton socks or stockings should be chosen. For adequate cleanliness socks should be changed daily.

6. Bathing.   Feet should be washed daily using plain (non-medicated) soap. Dry the feet carefully and gently especially the area between the toes.

7. Toe nails.   Nails should be trimmed so that the distal edge is straight. The corners of the nails must not be rounded. A nail file or clipper may be used.

If vision is impaired nails must only be treated by a chiropodist.

8. *Calluses and corns.*   These must be treated with great care because they represent the response of the skin to pressure or friction. They may be rubbed with an emery board or pumice stone if the physician and chiropodist concur.

No irritant chemicals may be used.

9. *Heat.*   A hot water bottle must never be placed against the skin of the feet.

No apology is necessary for repeating these simple instructions and no opportunity to reinforce them should be lost because despite these well recognized objectives many problems arise. These include the ability of the attendant, physician, nurse or chiropodist, to communicate the importance of the message. Further, the patient must be able to comprehend the instructions and be motivated to follow them. Motivation is greatest soon after the diabetes has been diagnozed but often a complacent attitude develops and the standard of care deteriorates as a result. Another opportunity is often provided following the first (hopefully minor) episode of infection or ulceration. Finally, the patient must have the physical capacity, e.g. eyesight and joint mobility, to care for himself and the social circumstances must be such that adequate care can be given. Unless all these elements — education, motivation and capacity to care for the feet are present, major difficulties will be encountered, as can be seen by the frequency with which patients present with major lesions. Some problems result from minor accidents in well motivated patients but there are a large group of patients who lack insight or the capacity to care for their feet and many intractable problems arise in this group.

Role of the chiropodist

The chiropodist is an essential member of the team which cares for diabetics and takes a major responsibility for the provision of this advice and support. The chiropodist fulfills several important roles:

Counselling.   A visit to the chiropodist may be less daunting for the patient than many visits to the doctor so that patients will often feel more relaxed and therefore more able to discuss their condition. The chiropodist should not lose any opportunity to advise the patient and particularly to warn against unsatisfactory footwear.

Treating minor lesions.   A small area of hyper-keratotis, an ingrowing toe nail or a small laceration may be trivial lesions in a foot with normal sensation and with a normal blood supply, but to a diabetic with an ischaemic, neuropathic foot such lesions are potentially disastrous because these apparently minor incidents can be followed by rapidly spreading infection or gangrene. The chiropodist will attempt to reduce the progression of these lesions and to advise the patient to consult the physician as soon as this becomes necessary. Much of the treatment to be described in the next section will carried out by the chiropodist.

MINOR LESIONS AND THEIR TREATMENT

The diabetic may suffer from all the foot conditions that a non-diabetic may incur. Only those lesions of special importance to diabetics are discussed in this section.

Lesions of the nails

These are discussed here because of their potential for causing serious problems. Like so many other aspects of the management of these patients the most important contribution to their care is the prevention of problems. The instructions to the patient regarding care of the nails have been mentioned above. If the nails are very thick or if the patient's eyesight or motor function are inadequate, care of the nails must be carried out by an attendant and this is usually the chiropodist.

Ingrowing toe nails

Infection or necrosis starting at the edge of an ingrowing toe nail has led to the amputation of many legs. This lesion which, in a normal foot, causes some discomfort and reduced mobility for a few days may, in an insensitive, ischaemic foot, be followed rapidly by spreading infection and necrosis. Any signs of infection around a toe nail must be regarded seriously and treated with rest and a full course of antibiotics (see p. 44). Evidence of necrosis (gangrene) is particularly sinister. The cause of the lesion known as an ingrowing toe nail is frequently improper cutting of the nail with the corners of the nail cut proximally and not left square (Fig. 7.2). A spur at the side of the nail breaks the epithelium adjacent to it and a chronic inflammatory reaction with granulation tissue formation is set up. This area provides a ready portal of entry for invasive organisms. The same result may follow the development of an excessively curved nail (Fig. 7.2). The weight-bearing forces tend to drive the edges of the nail through the skin and the same risk of infection follows.

The most important part of the management is the prevention of the lesion by adequate chiropody and counselling. Early lesions may be treated by gently lifting the edge of the nail and placing a small rolled piece of cotton wool beneath it. Excision of a triangular piece from the leading edge of the nail may reduce the tendency to lateral growth. The chiropodist may remove a narrow piece from the lateral edge which should include the offending splinter of nail. The sulcus should be packed with some wool soaked in mild antiseptic. This dressing should be changed regularly and reviewed at weekly intervals during the initial stages to ensure that the lateral spur does not form again. If these measures fail to control the ingrowth and the ankle pulses are present the nail may be removed (this

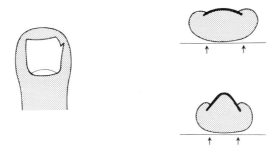

Fig. 7.2 (Left) The origin of an ingrowing toe nail. The right hand corner of the nail has been cut back leaving a small spur projecting. As the nail grows this spur penetrates the skin. (Right) Problems with an excessively curved nail. In the normal toe (above) weight-bearing forces flatten the nail. With a very curved nail (below) the vertical forces tend to drive the edges of the nail into the soft tissues of the toe.

should be carried out with general anaesthesia in these patients). Removal of the nail from an ischaemic foot is very hazardous and should seldom be carried out, and then only by a specialist because of the danger of spreading necrosis which might lead to an amputation. More extensive procedures such as removal of the nail bed are rarely necessary and are also specialist procedures in these patients.

Onychogryphosis

The development of thick curved nails (like a sheep's horn) is very common in elderly patients. The danger is that the thick hard nail will cause pressure and necrosis at its edges or, more commonly, on an adjacent toe. The small lesion which results may, like an ingrown toe nail, be the focus through which infection enters and the sequelae may be just as disastrous. Here also preventative treatment is important. The overgrowth must be removed so that the remaining nail cannot cause pressure on neighbouring toes. This can be achieved by regular abrasion which should, at least initially, be carried out by an expert.

Increased keratin formation

This is a normal response to increased pressure and friction on the skin and in normal feet there are areas where the keratin layer is thicker than in others. The presence of a localized increase in keratin should be regarded as indicating abnormal forces on the foot rather than an abnormal propensity in the diabetic to form keratin. The common sites involved are the sole of the foot in the region of the metatarsal heads, the lateral side of the fifth metatarsal base and the medial side of both the head of the first metatarsal and the region of the interphalangeal joint of the great toe. If the toes are clawed, friction on the inside of the shoe may cause callus formation over the proximal interphalangeal joint. A distinction is often made between a corn which forms over a non-weightbearing bony prominence and callus which forms over weightbearing surfaces. A corn may be a more sharply circumscribed lesion and usually has a core which may cause tenderness. However histologically the lesions are similar and they both arise from abnormal pressure or friction forces so that to make a rigid distinction between them seems artificial.

In the first instance treatment is directed to the removal of sources of trauma by the provision of adequate foot-wear and the local removal of hyperkeratoses. The role of the chiropodist in advising the patient regarding footwear has already been mentioned and this is the first and most important line of treatment. The callus may be removed by excision with a scalpel or by abrasion with emery boards or rotating burr (like a dentist's drill). The patient should be seen at regular intervals until the overgrowth of keratin has been controlled. Modification of the footwear is often required. Long-term treatment may be necessary because the predisposing cause, e.g. an underlying exostosis may remain. Chemical keratolytic agents should not be used and the patient must be discouraged from self-treatment with these materials because, if neuropathy is present, chemical damage to the skin may not be recognized by the patient.

If providing adequate shoes does not give sufficient relief from the hyperkeratosis, various methods for the relief of pressure may be tried. Simple but effective measures include keeping toes apart with small pieces of cotton wool and adhesive felt rings placed around the margins of a corn. Pads and plasters of various shapes may be used to relieve the pressure on the affected area by transferring it to adjacent areas. These may be purchased ready-made or cut to the desired pattern by the chiropodist. Great care must be taken that no new areas are endangered by these manoeuvres. For more difficult and extensive lesions, more elaborate appliances may be necessary (see section on Orthoses). Operative treatment to remove underlying bony prominences must never be undertaken unless it is certain that the blood supply to the foot is normal. These procedures have very little place in the management of a middle-aged diabetic population.

Ulcers on toes
The commonest site for an ulcer is over the dorsum of the interphalangeal joint in a patient with clawed toes. In these cases any device which reduces the depth of the shoe must be removed because the definitive treatment of these lesions is the relief of pressure or friction. Once adequate depth has been provided in the footwear the ulcer can be expected to heal. Ulcers of the tips of the toes (see Fig. 8.5) which occur at an earlier stage of clawing are usually self-curing: as the deformity increases the pressure on the affected area decreases. Interdigital ulcers are usually caused by pressure from an adjacent toe nail. They are treated by trimming the nail and keeping the toes apart by means of small cotton-wool dressings.

Plantar ulcers
If an ulcer develops during a period of observation it means that, for whatever reason, the preventative measures have failed. The ulcer has developed because the skin has been exposed to excessive stresses which have not been adequately controlled. A much more serious phase of the disease begins because there is now, in addition to the chances of continuing necrosis, a portal of entry for bacteria which may lead to the development of infection with more tissue destruction. A detailed assessment of the situation by physician and chiropodist must be undertaken as described in chapter 9. Many ulcers may continue to be managed on an Outpatient basis although much closer supervision will be needed.

The first sign that an ulcer has developed is the presence of some blood pigment in an area of thick callus. The floor of the ulcer may not be visible but the blood is a sure indication that the skin beneath has broken. As the callus is trimmed away, evidence of cavitation or necrossi is seen and finally the extent of the ulcer can be demonstrated. After passing the soft, soggy callus an area of granulation tissue which forms the floor of the ulcer can be seen. The keratin should be removed until the white callus has been removed and soft pink skin can be seen all around the ulcer. A large disposable scalpel blade is an appropriate instrument for this task. After cleaning with saline the ulcer should be covered with a piece of dry gauze which can be changed daily.

Relieving the pressure on the ulcerated area is the only way of allowing the ulcer to heal. This simple aim may be very difficult to achieve. The patient feels no pain and is able to walk normally so that it is often difficult to convince him that a major alteration in his lifestyle may be needed. Rest in bed is the ideal way of reducing the load and allowing the ulcer to heal. However this is usually not possible on economic grounds from the view of either the patient or of the hospital system. Appropriately designed insoles may relieve the pressure sufficiently so that healing can occur while the patient remains ambulant. Their design and fabrication is discussed on page 68. If possible, there should be a temporary decrease in weight-bearing for example by a period of rest in the afternoon.

Immobilization in a plaster cast is a form of treatment which is regularly used in third-world countries to treat severely ulcerated feet in patients with diabetes or leprosy because the patient is able to continue walking while healing occurs and therefore hospital beds are not required for the treatment of these patients. This method should probably be used more frequently although the excellent results obtained in communities where arterial disease is infrequent may not be easily obtainable in a Western community.

Like so many other situations in the management of these patients, this method requires meticulous care and rigorous attention to detail. The technique used by Brand will be described. Small pieces of padding are applied to the anterior surface of the tibia, to the malleoli and dorsal surface of the ankle joint. A single plaster bandage is applied from the region of the metatarsal heads to the upper tibia. This plaster is moulded to conform exactly to the contour of the leg and foot. If this is adequately achieved, there is no movement between limb and plaster so that friction injuries will not occur and the forces during walking are evenly distributed over as wide an area as possible. When this bandage is almost dry, sufficient extra plaster is added to make the cast rigid and a rubber 'heel' is added to allow weight-bearing. The cast may be removed after three or four weeks and the progress of healing reviewed.

The difficulties with this technique are largely related to the need for careful application of the plaster, remembering that the absence of pain sensation means that the patient will not complain of pain from developing plaster sores. Even when the ulcer is healed the problem is not over. The newly healed skin is very fragile and must be carefully protected. The sources of external pressure, which lead to the development of the ulcer, must be controlled and this will often require the combined attention of chiropodist, splintmaker and shoemaker. Finally, and this is often the most difficult part, the patient must understand that preventative measures will have to be continued for life.

FOOTWEAR AND PROSTHETICS

In the section on advice to the patient it has been pointed out that diabetics should never walk barefooted and the footwear worn should not cause trauma to the feet. The design of the footwear will depend on climate and culture, but the principles of protection and avoidance of injury are universal requirements. The routine instructions detailed (p. 60) can, if appropriately communicated and accepted, be very effective in reducing morbidity. However it is possible to define several groups of patients who have a high risk of development or progression of ulcers and these groups of patients require more specialized care. They are:

1. Patients with feet deformed by neuropathic change. The group most at risk are those with deformed feet as a result of changes in the joints of the foot. Considerable deformity can be produced which makes the wearing of conventional

shoes very difficult and unsafe. In other patients clawing of the toes which results from denervation of the small muscles of the foot sometimes produces a forefoot which can only be safely fitted in a shoe if the distance between sole and upper of the shoe is much greater than normal.

2. Patients with feet deformed as a result of operation. This may happen either because removal of a metatarsal head reduces the number of weight bearing points from 5 to 4, or because removal of a toe leaves neighbouring toes exposed. The possibility of removing these digits is discussed in Chapter 10.

3. Patients with plantar ulcers. In some patients with ulcers, after assessment as outlined in Chapter 9, it may be decided to treat the ulcer while allowing the patient to continue to walk. Patients who have recently healed plantar ulcers certainly require careful follow-up and many need modification of the footwear. There are several ways in which the footwear can be modified in order to meet the changed requirements of these patients.

Custom-built shoes
The provision of these shoes for many diabetics is beyond the financial resources of most communities and the craftsmen to make them are also in short supply. Shoes are time-consuming and expensive to produce and because the shape of the foot may be altered by operation a short time after the shoes are obtained, there is great potential for waste. Nevertheless in patients with grossly deformed feet the provision of special footwear is highly desirable. There may be available brands of ready-made shoes which have extra depth between the sole and the upper. This may allow the insertion of an insole and provide space so that clawed toes do not rub against the shoe. Specially made shoes must be made to comfortably enclose the foot. Extra depth to allow insertion of a 1 cm thick insole is often necessary. The appearance of the shoes must be as close as possible to that which is fashionable because shoes which are perceived by the patient as being ugly may be discarded.

The effect of different patterns of shoes on the distribution of forces under the foot was studied by Bauman et al (1963) using transducers beneath the foot as described on page 54. They studied patients whose neuropathy was due to leprosy and divided the subjects with anaesthetic feet into those with and without deformity. Those with deformity, which included the effects of repeated ulceration and loss of toes, were more closely related to the problem discussed here. There were two features in the design of the shoe which produced the greatest relief of load on the forefoot. They were (1) a rigid sole and (2) a rocker placed behind the area of the metatarsal heads. The effect of these devices is shown in Figure 7.3. During the step-off phase (see p. 50) when the load is normally concentrated on

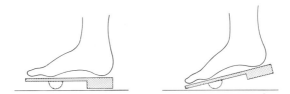

Fig. 7.3 Principles of a rocker shoe.

the metatarsal heads the effect of these modifications is to transfer part of the load to the area behind the metatarsal heads and away from the area which is most susceptible to the development of ulcers. Conventional shoes which are acceptable in appearance may be constructed incorporating these principles. The sole is made rigid by the insertion of a steel plate and the rocker bar may be added beneath the sole. Extra depth can be provided within the shoe for the addition of an insole if this is desired.

Insoles

Appliances which reduce the space available within the shoe must be used with extreme caution. A pad beneath the metatarsal heads may have some place in reducing the deformity of clawed toes, but it must only be used if the metatarsophalangeal and interphalangeal joints are still mobile. If the joints are stiff, the appliance will not reduce the deformity and will increase the damage by causing pressure between the dorsum of the interphalangeal joints and the shoe. Evidence of increased pressure such as hyperkeratosis or reddening, must be very carefully sought if this device is used. Insoles are especially useful in patients whose feet have been deformed by operation or who have plantar ulcers. They may be used to protect exposed toes or to relieve pressure on particular areas of the foot. The polyethylene plastic, Plastazote, is a suitable material. It differs from a sponge in that the air pockets do not communicate with each other and it can be moulded when heated to 140°C. Figure 7.4 shows the design of a splint to lessen the pressure on the area of the second and third metatarsal heads. It is made from two pieces of material each 6 mm thick. An outline of the foot is traced on a sheet of Plastazote and the design of the second piece, shown shaded in the diagram, is drawn. The smaller piece is cut so that only one thickness of material lies beneath the area of the foot from which it is desired to relieve pressure. The smaller piece is placed in position and both are put on a sheet of paper and heated in the oven. They have been adequately heated when they feel sticky to the palpating fingers. The two pieces will adhere when heated and the foot can be placed on the material as it cools but is still warm enough to mould. The foot is placed on the position originally outlined. A block of Plastazote approximately 20 mm thick should be placed on the floor beneath the splint. The edges of the splint can be trimmed to fit the shoe. If a mistake is made during this process the Plastazote will regain its original shape after it is reheated in the oven. An alternative method is to use a

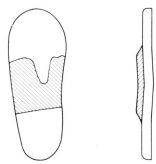

Fig. 7.4 Design of a Plastazote splint to relieve pressure on the heads of the second and third metatarsal bones.

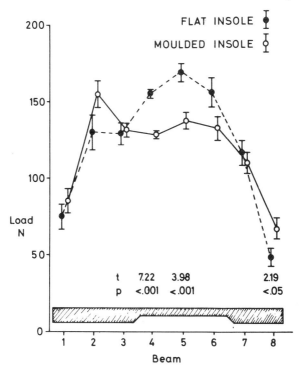

Fig. 7.5 Effect of wearing the splint shown in Fig. 7.4. There was a significant reduction in load in the area where the splint was thinnest (shown by the shaded area at the bottom of the figure).

single piece 12 mm thick. This will even out the distribution of load across the forefoot but probably does not produce the same reduction in load as the method described. Further sculpturing of the insole may be carried out with a knife or razor blade to produce greater relief from pressure in a desired area.

After the splint has been worn for several hours the shoes and stockings must be removed and the feet, especially the toes, inspected for signs of abnormal pressure. It may be washed weekly in warm water and mild detergent and can be expected to last 6–8 weeks of daily use. At the end of this time, the splint can be replaced or renewed by attaching a new piece of Plastazote beneath it. Figure 7.5 shows the effect of wearing this splint when tested on the apparatus described in Chapter 6. The reduction in load obtained, about 20% of the force under the designated area, is likely to be sufficiently great that it is clinically useful.

This material may also be used to make a device which provides protection for exposed toes. Figure 7.6 shows a patient who developed an ulcer on the tip of the second toe which had been left exposed after removal of the great toe. A splint was constructed to protect the toes and the ulcer subsequently healed. The gap left by the removal of the great toe was filled by several pieces of Plastazote which were stuck together after heating their surfaces with a soldering iron. The piece covering the toes was similarly attached. Plastazote has also been used to make sandals and shoes which have been advocated in the treatment of patients with similar foot disorders particularly the deformities resulting from leprosy and rheumatoid arthritis.

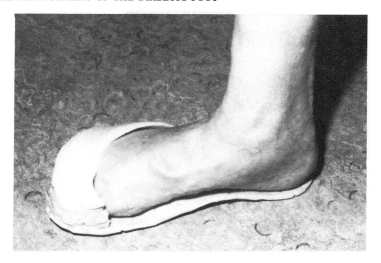

Fig. 7.6 Splint designed to protect the remaining toes after removal of the great toe. The toes are covered by a thin piece of Plastazote.

There are several other ways in which the problem of redistributing the load under the foot might be approached. Clearly a method which allows the patient to continue normal activities while an ulcer heals is of great psychological and financial benefit. One method involves using the principle that water transmits pressure equally in all directions. Preliminary testing has indicated that this method may be effective. Part of the sole of a shoe was cut away and a bag containing water was inserted. Testing of this device clearly showed that there was a reduction in the peak loads carried. The problem not yet solved is to contain the water in a material which is strong enough to withstand the repetitive forces produced by walking for a long period.

The devices described in this section may be of benefit to individual patients. Their design and fabrication requires much time and attention to detail but the potential rewards are great.

REFERENCES

Bauman J H, Girling J P, Brand P W 1963 Plantar pressures and trophic ulceration. Journal of Bone and Joint Surgery 45B: 652–673.
Brandaleone H, Standard S, Ralli E P 1937 Prophylactic foot treatment in patients with diabetes mellitus. Annals of Surgery 105: 120–124.
Brooks A P, Nairn I M, Baird J D 1980 Changes in glycosolated haemoglobin after poor control in insulin dependent diabetics. British Medical Journal 281: 707–710
Cahill G F, Etzwiler D D, Freinkel N 1976 "Control" and diabetes. The New England Journal of Medicine 294: 1004–1005
Chazan B I, Balodimos M C, Ryan J R, Marble A 1970 Twenty-five to forty-five years of diabetes with and without vascular complications. Diabetologia 6: 565–569
Koenig R G, Cerami A 1980 Haemoglobin A$_{Ic}$ and diabetes mellitus. Annual Review of Medicine 31: 29–34
Siperstein M D, Foster D W, Knowles H C, Levine R, Madison L L, Roth J 1977 Control of blood glucose and diabetic vascular disease. New England Journal of Medicine 296: 1060–1063
Tchobroutsky G 1978 Relation of diabetic control to development of microvascular complications. Diabetologia 15: 143–152

8

Clinical features of major lesions

Despite the efforts of patient and attendants, major lesions may develop. It is the purpose of this chapter to describe the ways in which these patients present. All too often, patients come for treatment with a foot which has been swollen and discharging for a period of days or weeks. These patients will usually notice, if they test the urine, that the amount of glycosuria has increased. At this stage admission to hospital will be necessary and will probably be followed by one or more operations, a prolonged period of immobility and possible loss of a major part of the foot or limb. On the other hand, many minor lesions can be managed or prevented from extending by provision of adequate footwear and careful chiropody (Ch. 7).

THE VULNERABLE FOOT

A foot in which arterial disease or neuropathy or both are present is liable to develop major complications. The effects of arterial disease and neuropathy have been described in Chapters 3 and 4 respectively, and the detailed presenting features are given below. However, it is helpful to summarize the clinical findings in a foot in which the conditions for the development of a major lesion exist. Detailed assessment is discussed in Chapter 9.

Evidence of ischaemia
    a history of intermittent claudication or rest pain
    coldness of the foot
    absence of ankle pulses
    dependent rubor
Standard textbooks often provide a longer list of features but those given here will enable a useful clinical assessment to be made.

Evidence of neuropathy
    the posture of the foot
        clawing of the toes
        callus over pressure areas
        deformity due to neuropathic changes in joints
    on palpation the foot feels dry and also warm if the blood supply is sufficient
    loss of light touch and pain (pin prick) sensation on the toes and foot. In more
    severe cases this sensory loss may extend to the calf

loss of perception of vibration on the foot, at the ankle and perhaps at the knee
absence of ankle tendon reflexes and perhaps patellar tendon reflexes.

Evidence of previous episodes
Any patient who has had an ulcer or amputation of a toe or part of the foot has a
high risk of developing further problems.

A patient with one or more of these groups of features must be very carefully
supervised and may need the provision of special footwear as described in Chapter 7. Many patients are able to avoid the development of major lesions but it is
from this population that the difficult problems of assessment and management
will occur.

The following sections describe the common modes of presentation of major lesions of the foot. This listing is not exclusive and represents a simplification because combinations of lesions frequently occur. However it is helpful to consider
these principal ways in which the patients present.

GANGRENE

There are three major groups of patients who present with macroscopic areas of
dead tissue.

Gangrene of toes
The lesion often starts from a minor injury, e.g. while cutting the toenail,
although in many cases the initial lesion was not recognized. This wound fails to
heal, the skin edges become black and the gangrene spreads to involve the whole
of the toe. Adjacent toes may also become gangrenous. There is often a clear de-
marcation between the dead and living tissues (dry gangrene) although the gangrene may gradually progress to involve the foot (Fig. 8.1). This lesion is due to

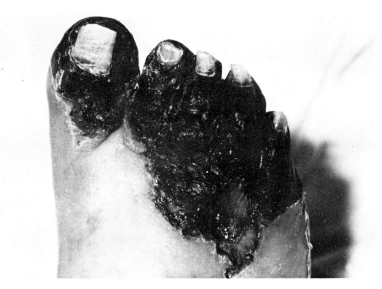

Fig. 8.1 Ischaemic gangrene of foot

atherosclerotic occlusion of arteries. There will be no ankle pulses palpable, and the foot and lower leg will be cold. Ischaemic rest pain will be present if there is not severe neuropathy. The pain may have preceded the development of gangrene.

Gangrenous patches

1. Areas of gangrene may occur on parts of the foot which are exposed to pressure. The common sites are the heel, the malleoli and the areas of the first metatarsal head medially and the base of the fifth metatarsal. They may vary from a few millimetres to several centimetres in diameter. They typically occur in bedridden patients who have severe atherosclerosis but neuropathy is frequently present so that the lesions do not cause pain. They usually remain about the same size and sometimes slowly heal.

2. Small areas of gangrene may occur on parts of the foot not subject to pressure because of embolism of atheromatous debris. Small infarcts in the skin result. There are usually multiple areas 2–3 mm in diameter in several parts of the toes and foot (Fig. 8.2). These are a purple-blue colour and do not blanch on pressure. They are usually painful and may heal beneath a small scab or eschar which forms on the skin. These lesions are atherosclerotic in origin and not specific to diabetics. The large arteries are usually patent (otherwise the emboli would not have reached the skin) and the debris may be thrombus arising from an aneurysm, e.g. of the aorta or femoral artery or debris from an atherosclerotic plaque in any proximal artery. Occasionally the areas of necrosis are so large that amputation of a toe is required.

3. Bullous lesions. These are often superficial blisters which heal rapidly but deeper lesions which result in areas of skin necrosis can occur (Hadden and Allen 1969).

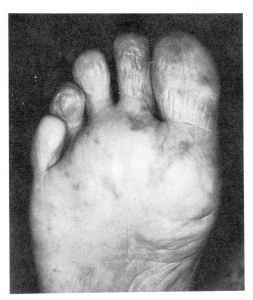

Fig. 8.2 Areas of ischaemic skin from occlusion of small vessels with atheromatous debris. (This patient was not diabetic)

Gangrene with infection

Dead tissue is always contaminated with bacteria. However in most patients with gangrene as described above, invasive infection does not occur. There are three situations in which gangrene and invasive infection occur together. Two are described here and the third, anaerobic cellulitis, is described in the section on Infection (p. 78).

a. Spreading atherosclerotic gangrene. This begins as outlined in 1. above. If infection follows, it may spread (wet gangrene) through tissue which because of a poor blood supply, is unable to confine the process so that further necrosis occurs. This type of gangrene is a threat to life because spreading anaerobic cellulitis may follow. This type of infection is the dangerous outcome of conservative treatment of gangrene although such a policy is often justified by the age and general condition of the patient. Wet gangrene occurs in non-diabetics as well as in diabetics.

b. Gangrene in a well vascularised foot (Fig. 8.3). This is one of the characteristic lesions in diabetics and is sometimes labelled 'diabetic gangrene'. It is distinguished from the gangrene described in 1 above because it develops rapidly and is almost painless because of the presence of severe neuropathy. It may start in an identical manner to atherosclerotic gangrene, e.g. from a minor wound on a toe. Necrosis may extend because the infection causes thrombosis of digital vessels and signs of deep infection in the foot are usually present. The foot is warm and ankle pulses can be felt if they are not masked by oedema. Often attention is drawn to the foot by the smell from the infected tissue rather than by pain. The necrosis may involve extensive areas, e.g. several toes and the adjacent part of the foot.

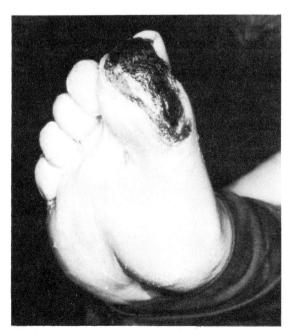

Fig. 8.3 Gangrene in a well vascularised foot. In this case gangrene followed wearing a new pair of shoes. Both ankle pulses were present.

ULCERS

Plantar ulcers

This is the characteristic neuropathic foot lesion of the diabetic. Synonyms include trophic or penetrating ulcer and mal perforans. They are typically painless and occur over areas which normally carry weight or which, because of structural changes, have come to carry excessive weight. The mechanisms by which they develop have been discussed in Chapter 7 (p. 65). The earliest changes are an area of hyper-keratosis often over a metatarsal head. The keratin may be several millimetres thick at its centre. If uncontrolled, eventually a small area of dark staining will appear in the keratin. This material, which is altered blood, indicates that the epithelium beneath has been breached. If the excess keratin is pared away a small ulcer will be found. At this stage the ulcer is often no more than a linear split in the skin. If the area of pressure is unrelieved, the ulcer will enlarge, often reaching 1–2 cm diameter (Fig. 8.4). As the necrosis extends laterally it also extends to involve the deeper tissues of the foot, progressively involving aponeurosis, tendon sheath and bone. Infection may occur at any stage and may spread along tendon sheaths or other planes opened up by the extension of the ulcer. In a deformed foot, e.g. following neuropathic degeneration of the tarsal joints, ulcers may develop over the resulting bony prominences. The base of the ulcer is scarred and thickened. These ulcers are notoriously resistant to treatment if walking continues.

In these patients signs of neuropathy will be detectable. Diminution or absence of the perception of pain is almost always present. The circulation to the foot may range from normal to severely impaired. The complications of these ulcers are progressive tissue necrosis and infection. The non-operative management of these

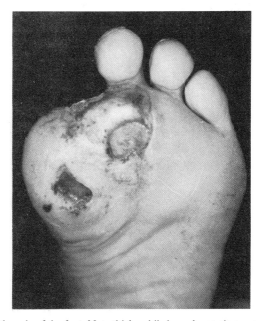

Fig. 8.4 Two ulcers on the sole of the foot. Note thick, while hyperkeratotic areas.

ulcers has been discussed in the previous chapter. The indications for and details of operative treatment are given in Chapter 10.

Ulcers of the toes

The commonest site is on the dorsum of the proximal interphalangeal joint of a clawed toe. These toes, because they are raised dorsally beyond the plane of the foot, are often rubbed by the inside of the shoe. Hyperkeratosis or inflammation may precede the breakdown of the skin and the development of a small ulcer. If the blood supply to the foot is impaired, such an ulcer may initiate the development of gangrene as outlined above. If infection becomes established in the ulcer, it may result in gangrene or spread to the deep tissues of the foot.

Ulcers may develop on the tips of the toes (Fig. 8.5). This occurs during the early stages of clawing when the tips of the toes still make contact with the ground. Pressure from adjacent toes or toenails may also cause ulcers. They occur commonly on the lateral side of the third or fourth toes due to pressure from the fourth or fifth toe respectively. These ulcers are usually painless but they may be quite deep and of course they present a portal of entry for infection.

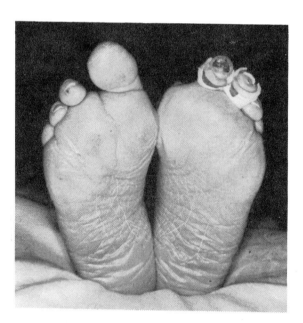

Fig. 8.5 Ulcers on tips of clawed toes.

INFECTION

The diagnosis of infection is made difficult because of the loss of one of the cardinal symptoms of infection, pain. The diabetic is liable to the whole range of infections which affect non-diabetics. These include the non-specific bacterial infection as well as the specific mycotic infections which are particularly common in tropical climates.

There are two forms of infection which are particularly important in diabetics:

Deep infection

Because of the absence of pain, the presence and extent of these infections is often underestimated. Although the severe throbbing pain associated with an abscess is not present, there is often a dull ache or burning or tingling sensation reported. There is often pus discharging through a sinus or ulcer which preceded the infection. The discharge of pus can be produced by pressure over the mid part of the sole or by moving an infected joint (Fig. 8.6). The most important signs are swelling and redness (Fig. 8.7). This may be seen in the dorsum of the web spaces of the foot because many of the lymphatics from the superficial tissues drain in this direction. Swelling of the toes may also be a useful sign. However the most characteristic sign is separation of the toes due to diffuse oedema of the deep tissues of the foot, and this almost always means that there is pus deep in the foot. The thickness of the plantar fascia masks swelling of the anterior part of the sole of the foot but swelling and redness may be seen inferior and posterior to the medial malleolus. This is because the infection commonly tracks along the flexor tendon sheaths which pass behind the medial malleolus. These sheaths also provide the route by which infection may spread into the lower part of the leg. Any of these signs indicates that the patient should be admitted to hospital.

A localized abscess may also form on the dorsum of the foot. Infection here follows a lesion on a toe. Swelling is very common in this site because the subcutaneous tissue is relatively loose and the lymphatics run through this area. The

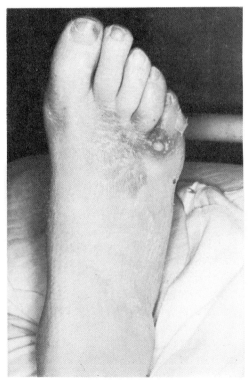

Fig. 8.6 Infection presenting on dorsal aspect of foot from a plantar ulcer which had involved the fifth metatarsaophalangeal joint.

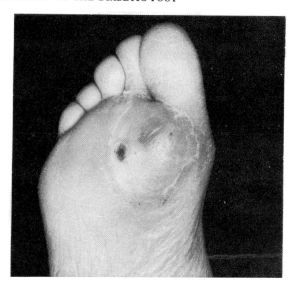

Fig. 8.7 Cellulitis in foot from an unrecognized drawing-pin through the sole of the shoe. Drainage was not required

sign of fluctuation may be difficult to detect because the pus may be deep to the extensor tendons. A small collection of pus is frequently found here when deep infections of the sole of the foot are being drained, e.g. by a ray amputation (see page 104). In the most severe cases there will be swelling and redness in the calf indicating that the infection has spread to that region. Once this stage has been reached it is likely that the foot will be lost.

Anaerobic infections

These are very dangerous because of the rapidity with which they spread and cause a systemic infection.

Ischaemia of the tissues is an important predisposing factor. They may occur in any foot in which the skin has been broken but they are particularly likely to occur following surgery, e.g. local amputation. Fortunately most of the infections with anaerobic bacteria, e.g. bacteroides species, remain localized. There are two forms of spreading anaerobic infection:

Clostridial

This infection is identical to that occurring in non-diabetics. The classical form is a spreading myositis in which the patient has evidence of severe generalized infection with a high fever and leucocytosis. Less often there may be a spreading subcutaneous infection in which gas is present in the subcutaneous tissue but where the skin appears relatively healthy until late in the disease. Gram-positive spore-forming bacilli will be seen in a smear from the affected tissue and sometimes, shortly before death, in a smear from the peripheral blood.

Non-clostridial

The features of non-clostridial gas gangrene in diabetics have been described by

Bird et al (1977). They include the insidious onset, absence of pain and the late appearance of skin necrosis and crepitus. This discussion has concentrated on the presentation of major foot lesions almost all of which will require treatment as an inpatient in hospital. Other problems have been discussed earlier in the book including minor infections (page 42), problems with the nails (page 63), and deformities of the foot (page 66).

REFERENCES

Bird D, Giddings A E B, Jones S M 1977 Non-clostridial gas gangrene in the diabetic lower limb. Diabetologia 13: 373–376
Hadden D R, Allen G E 1969 Bullous lesions in the feet of diabetic patients. Diabetologia 5: 422

9

Assessment of the patient with a foot lesion

Vascular disease and neuropathy set the scene for the development of complications. Infection, which may be so important in causing tissue damage, follows some breach in the skin which either passes unrecognized due to neuropathy or fails to heal because of an impaired arterial supply. In considering the development of foot lesions, arterial disease and neuropathy must be regarded as developing and progressing independently, despite the possible role of arterial disease as a cause of neuropathy. This means that patients are encountered with all possible combinations: from extensive arterial disease and no detectable neuropathy, to severe neuropathy and no detectable arterial disease. Most commonly both will be present and the aim of assessment is to determine the contribution made by each.

A gangrenous or ulcerated limb is not an immediate threat to life unless a severe infection (particularly anaerobic cellulitis) supervenes. This means that in most cases there is time to make a careful assessment of both the general condition of the patient and the state of the foot. The development of a serious foot lesion is a major event in the natural history of the diabetes and provides an opportunity for a detailed assessment of the situation, particularly with regard to the development of complications of the diabetes. After this assessment and the treatment of life-threatening complications, the likely outcome of the episode must be considered. The two extreme outcomes are that the lesion will heal or that a major amputation will be needed. In between are the possibilities that reconstructive surgery or a minor amputation may be necessary. Firm decisions cannot be made before a detailed review has been made of the general and local condition.

The majority of patients can be successfully assessed by standard clinical techniques and simple laboratory tests. There is no doubt, however, that the difficulties of making precise assessments cause mistakes to be made.

A variety of methods, of greater or lesser complexity, are available to provide additional information and the value and limitations of these measurements will be discussed.

GENERAL ASSESSMENT

Control of diabetes
The state of the diabetic control must be assessed. The urine is examined for sugar and ketones and the blood glucose level determined. The problems of assess-

ing the medium to long-term control of the diabetes have been discussed on page 58. The urgency of regaining control of the diabetes will depend on the severity of the foot lesion but in the more severe cases it will be necessary to substitute injections of regular insulin for the patient's usual regimen. See Appendix for details.

Presence of complications of diabetes.
In patients who have been under regular review this knowledge will be available, but the development of a major complication provides an opportunity to undertake a more detailed assessment.

Retinopathy
The visual acuity should be tested and the optic fundi examined. Visual impairment may seriously prejudice the ability of the patient to care adequately for the foot. More detail, if desired, can be obtained by fluorescein angiography which will demonstrate areas of ischaemia which cannot be detected by other methods.

Renal function
Qualitatitive and quantitative measurement of the degree of proteinuria should be carried out. Blood urea and creatinine estimation will give more detailed information regarding the degree of impairment of renal function. Renal failure is one of the important causes of death of these patients and once proteinuria occurs there is usually a progressive, although thankfully often, slow deterioration in renal function. Infection, ischaemia and papillary necrosis are important lesions which may aggravate the renal failure.

Cardiac disease
The history will give details of past episodes of myocardial infarction or cardiac failure. An electrocardiogram may give evidence of ischaemia or conduction defect which was not detected by physical examination. This information is important in determining the fitness of the patient for any operation which may be contemplated.

Social factors
The care that can be given depends to a large extent on the socio-economic circumstances. The problems encountered in caring for patients in an affluent Western society are very different from those in less wealthy communities. On an individual level the patient's home circumstances are important. Successful outpatient treatment and the prevention of recurrent lesions depends very much on the ability of the patient to co-operate in the treatment plan. The availability of domiciliary nursing services and the health of the husband or wife of the patient can have a great influence on the outcome. In this regard there are a group of patients with neuropathy, usually men between 50–70, often with a high alcohol intake, who have very little insight into the potential seriousness of their condition and who are unable to achieve the standard of personal care necessary for control of the condition. The morbidity and mortality are high in this group.

LOCAL ASSESSMENT

This is directed at determining the severity of infection, arterial disease and neuropathy. The presence and severity of infection determines the urgency with which treatment must be undertaken. Once this has been established the major part of the assessment will be to decide the relative severity of arterial disease and neuropathy. It is very important to remember that the severity of the arterial disease will be the major determinant of healing.

Infection

Infection may vary in severity from a small area of redness around a bunion to a life-threatening spreading anaerobic cellulitis. Early diagnosis and control of infection is very important in the management of these patients. Invasive infection must be treated vigorously to prevent spread which will inevitably lead to further loss of tissue. Redness of the skin may result from friction or developing ischaemic necrosis. If the skin is intact, attention should be directed to relieving the source of injury. However if the skin is broken and there is surrounding inflammation, it is usually wise to assume that there is infection occurring and treat with antibiotics. Any open wound or ulcer will be contaminated with bacteria and presents a portal through which infection may become established, although invasive infection will not necessarily occur. It is important to distinguish between contaminated and infected wounds because the former require careful observation but the latter require aggressive chemotherapy. The immediately dangerous infections are spreading anaerobic sepsis, which is a serious threat to life, and the presence of a deep abscess, which causes progressive tissue damage. The features of these infections have been described on page 78.

The presence of general features of infection will depend on the amount of tissue involved and the presence of pus. High fever and marked leucocytosis will indicate the presence of an abscess — usually deep in the foot. An increased tendency to hyperglycaemia and ketosis is also indirect evidence of uncontrolled infection.

Radiology of the foot

Radiographs of the foot should be taken if there is any suspicion of infection deep in the foot, e.g. abscess or osteomyelitis. The signs which will suggest the presence of osteomyelitis are:

1. Bone destruction. In these patients this is commonly seen at a metatarsophalangeal joint or in the inter-phalangeal joint of the great toe. In the earlier cases these will be small erosions at the margins of the bone; later there is obvious destruction of the articulating surfaces.

2. Sequestrum formation and subperiosteal new bone may be seen but are uncommon in these patients.

3. Gas in the tissues. A small amount of gas may be seen along the track between an ulcer and an underlying joint. Gas may also be seen in an abscess cavity in the foot. Large amounts of subcutaneous gas, especially if it extends towards the leg, indicate the presence of a serious anaerobic infection.

4. Soft tissue swelling may often be seen due to the inflammation which accompanies inflammation.

The changes of bone destruction described above may appear identical to the changes which accompany neuropathic degeneration in the metatarsophalangeal joint region. These findings have been described in Chapter 4, where the difficulty in distinguishing neuropathic from infective changes was pointed out. If there is clinical evidence of infection in the foot, evidence of bone destruction should be assumed to be due to infection. The same conclusion should be reached if a communication between a joint and an ulcer can be demonstrated by gentle probing or if tendon is visible in the base of an ulcer. Radiological signs of neuropathic degeneration between the tarsal joints are unlikely to influence the outcome of infection or ulcer in the forefoot. There are several radiological signs of accompanying arterial disease. In severe ischaemia there may be a generalized osteoporosis in the bones of the foot. In addition, calcification of the metatarsal or digital vessels is commonly seen (Fig. 9.1, 9.2). It is not necessary to take special soft tissue radiographs to search for this because these changes, although they reflect prolonged hyperglycaemia, do not indicate the presence of arterial disease which will impair healing of foot lesions.

Arterial disease

Presence of pain

If the nerve supply to the foot is intact, ulcers and gangrene are painful. The absence of pain means that there is neuropathy present but gives no indication of the severity of the arterial disease. On the other hand, ischaemic rest pain means that there is major artery obstruction present. The features of this pain are quite

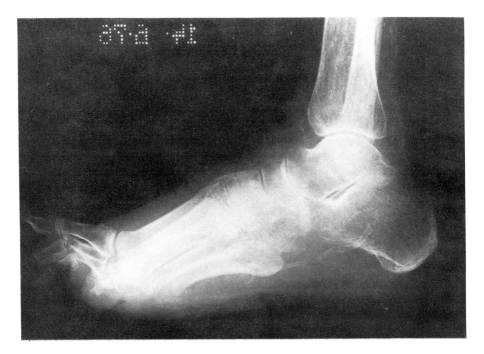

Fig. 9.1 Calcification of arteries. Extensive calcification of the posterior tibial artery and its terminal branches. Same patient as Fig. 3.7

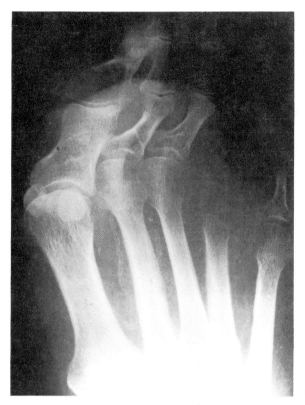

Fig. 9.2 Calcification of metatarsal arteries. Calcification to this extent is commonly seen in the feet of diabetics

characteristic. It occurs at rest (in contrast to ischaemic exercise pain or intermittent claudication which, by definition, occurs only on exercise). In its mildest forms the patient may complain only of coldness and numbness of the toes at night and this symptom may be difficult to distinguish from the symptoms of peripheral neuropathy. In more severe cases the patient has a constant, nagging, severe pain in the toes and foot. The pain is worse when the patient is recumbent and may be eased by hanging the leg over the side of the bed or walking on the cold floor. The patient may only be able to sleep by sitting in a chair with the legs dependent. This last feature distinguishes ischaemic pain from pain associated with infection because pain due to infection is relieved by elevation of the limb.

Palpation of pulses
If the ankle pulses are palpable there is enough blood reaching the foot to allow a local amputation to heal. In general, the need for a below-the-knee or higher amputation in such a patient represents a therapeutic disaster. The presence of one or other of the dorsalis pedis and posterior tibial pulses means that either the axial arterial system is patent or there are very well developed collateral vessels.

If the pulses are impalpable it means that either there is arterial obstruction or there may be so much oedema of the foot that normal arteries are impalpable. The pulses higher in the leg should be examined. If the popliteal pulse is absent, but the femoral pulse is present, the superficial femoral artery is obstructed. However, this does not necessarily mean that arterial obstruction is the cause of the lesion or that local amputation will fail. There may be sufficient collateral circulation to maintain the viability of the foot and even to allow local healing to occur although the time taken for wounds to heal is likely to be prolonged. If the popliteal pulse is present then the femoral artery is patent, although it may be stenosed. In these circumstances, if major arteries are obstructed the site of occlusion must be distal to the popliteal arteries. The implication is that arterial reconstruction is unlikely to be practicable. Thus although inexperienced observers often find the popliteal pulse difficult to feel, it is a sign of great importance in these patients. The presence of a popliteal pulse and the absence of both ankle pulses is a situation which seldom occurs in non-diabetic subjects because obstruction to the vessels below the knee is relatively uncommon in non-diabetics.

If the femoral pulse is absent, more distal pulses are unlikely to be present. This situation which indicates the presence of obstruction to the iliac arteries is relatively uncommon in diabetics. Figure 9.3 provides a summary of these findings.

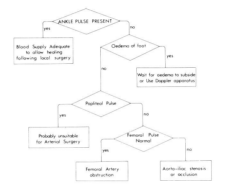

Fig. 9.3 Flow-chart for findings on palpation of pulses

Temperature of the skin
Feeling the temperature of the skin may be a good guide to the adequacy of the circulation to the limb: coldness is an important sign of ischaemia. In patients with femoral artery obstruction there is often a distinct change in temperature of the skin at the level of mid-point of the tibia. In addition the skin over the knee on the affected side may be warmer because of the presence of subcutaneous collateral vessels. A cold foot with a temperature gradient at mid-tibia suggests a femoral artery obstruction producing moderate to severe ischaemia. If there is obstruction above the origin of the profunda femoris artery the temperature gradient may be at mid-thigh level.

Classification of the patients on the basis of the temperature of the skin of the foot can provide a useful basis for determining the likely success of local amputation (Williams et al 1974).

The importance of areas of increased warmth in indicating areas which are inflamed as the result of repetitive mechanical trauma has been mentioned on page 57.

Neuropathy

A detailed clinical examination of the central and peripheral nervous system should be undertaken. The possible findings can be inferred from the discussion in Chapter 4. They include changes in pupillary reactions, cranial nerve lesions, evidence of neuropathy involving the upper limbs especially mononeuropathies and evidence of proximal muscle wasting associated with the syndrome of amyotrophy.

Examination of the foot and leg will reveal the majority of the signs. Inspection of the posture of the foot is very important. Clawing of the toes, especially if accompanied by thinning of the plantar fat pad so that the metatarsal heads are more prominent, suggests that there is neuropathy affecting the small muscles of the foot. Local areas of hyperkeratosis may be followed by painless plantar ulcers which are a characteristic result of diabetic neuropathy. Ulcers may be present at other sites of pressure, e.g. the interphalangeal joint of the great toe, the base of the fifth metatarsal and the dorsum of interphalangeal joints of clawed toes. The absence of dark necrotic tissue is typical. The deformity produced by neuropathic joints is usually seen in the region of the intertarsal joints. This may result in a deformity which is so disabling that the patient may not be able to wear ordinary shoes. Neuropathic change involving the metatarsal bones will only be detected on X-ray. Warmth of the skin of the foot implies an adequate blood supply, with or without infection and autonomic neuropathy.

Sensory testing, particularly for light touch and pin prick, should be performed. In the presence of a plantar ulcer there will be decreased perception of pain in the toes and forefoot. Loss of vibration sense at the ankle is very common. This sense is also lost in non-diabetic elderly patients and this sign alone does not indicate the presence of diabetic neuropathy. However, loss of vibration sense at the knee or higher levels is definitely abnormal.

Changes in the tendon reflexes occur in parallel with the severity of the neuropathy. Loss of the ankle reflex accompanies loss of vibration sense at the ankle as part of the ageing process, and this sign is not of major significance. Loss of the patellar tendon reflex indicates moderately severe neuropathy.

The function of the small muscles of the foot is difficult to test clinically, although its presence can be inferred from the postural changes described above, and can be demonstrated easily by electrophysiological testing. Weakness of the movements of the ankle and toes, which indicates a more severe neuropathy, can be demonstrated in about half the patients with lesions. Occasionally the patient will have foot drop from a mononeuropathy involving the common peroneal nerve. The presence of autonomic neuropathy may be detected easily at the bedside by observing the fall in blood pressure which occurs when the subject stands up from a lying position. The more detailed tests of autonomic function have been described in Chapter 4.

At the end of the examination an assessment must be made of the relative severity of infection, ischaemia and neuropathy. This can often be done adequately by the standard clinical examination outlined above, but on many occasions there remain doubts, particularly about the adequacy of the blood supply. The tests which may be used to provide more information are the subject of the next section.

SPECIAL TESTS

The assessment discussed above is obtained using standard clinical methods: this section discusses additional investigations which may be performed. Some of these tests, e.g. Doppler ultrasound, radionuclide scanning and angiography will be available in most general hospitals. Others, although often simple in concept, will only be used in centres with special interests or where research projects are being undertaken. In each case, the author's opinion of the usefulness and applicability of the methods is given.

The tests to be described in this section are all concerned with the circulation to the limb. This is because it is the adequacy of the blood supply which is the major determinant of healing of any wound or ulcer. The tests can be grouped into those used for measuring arterial blood pressure and those which study radioisotope perfusion or clearance. Special tests are available for studying the functions of both the autonomic and somatic parts of the nervous system. The changes in nerve conduction have been described on page 27 and the tests which may be used to test autonomic function are given on pages 30–33. The tests for somatic neuropathy do not provide any information which might be useful in establishing the short term prognosis although the persistence of neuropathy may, of course, be an important factor in determining the development of subsequent lesions.

Measurement of blood pressure

The ability to measure the arterial blood pressure in the legs has had a major impact on the practice of vascular surgery. Several techniques will be discussed. They all rely on the detection of returning blood flow distal to a cuff which is being deflated from suprasystolic levels, and are identical in principle to the palpatory method for measuring brachial artery pressure. They are of considerable benefit because they allow the measurement of blood pressure with acceptable accuracy over the whole range from normal to less than 20 mm mercury. This allows a quantitative assessment of the severity of the arterial disease to be made because the level of the systolic pressure measured at the ankle relates well to the clinical state of the patient (Yao 1970).

The sensitivity of the assessment can be increased if exercise or some other hyperaemic stimulus is applied before the pressure is measured. If there is significant arterial stenosis, a fall in pressure at the ankle will occur after exercise and this is the basis of a widely-used screening test for patients with vascular disease. Before these tests were available the assessment of the patient by physical examination depended largely on the ability to feel the ankle pulses. This sign is very susceptible to variation between observers and the pulses may be masked by the presence of oedema. In addition, although the pulses are absent the leg may be symptomless. It is the author's view that the use of one of these tests is an essential part of the practice of vascular surgery.

Doppler ultrasound

If a continuous beam of sound is transmitted through tissues it will be reflected from various objects in its path. If these objects are moving, e.g. blood cells, the

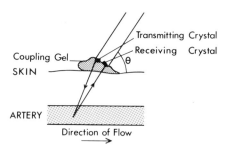

Fig. 9.4 Doppler principle. The frequency shift of the returning sound depends on the transmitted frequency, the angle between the beam and the moving particles and the velocity of the particles.

frequency of the reflected wave will be altered and this change will be proportional to the velocity of movement (Fig. 9.4). This is the basis of the Doppler ultrasound method. The apparatus consists of a probe, which contains both transmitting receiving elements, connected to a box which generates the ultrasound and processes the returning waves. These are manipulated electronically to produce a signal which may be fed either to a speaker to produce an audible output or a chart recorder to produce a visible tracing. The main use of this apparatus is to act as a very sensitive pulse detector. It can be used over arteries as large as the femoral arteries and as small as the digital arteries (at least in the fingers). Signals from intra-abdominal arteries are usually distorted by reflections from overlying loops of bowel. From tracings of the blood flow velocity patterns, the state of the proximal arteries may be inferred but this application is not sufficiently sensitive to justify its widespread use for this purpose. The most common application is in the measurement of arterial systolic blood pressure. The probe is placed over an artery distal to an occluding cuff, and the pressure at which the signal returns during deflation of the cuff from suprasystolic levels is taken as the systolic blood pressure. It is most valuable in measuring the pressure in the arteries low in the leg. The occluding cuff is applied to the lower part of the calf, and the probe is placed over the posterior tibial artery behind the medial malleolus and the dorsalis pedis artery over the metatarsal bones. If the dorsalis pedis artery is absent, a signal from the terminal branch of the peroneal artery can usually be heard more laterally on the dorsum of the foot. The systolic pressure should be recorded from both the posterior tibial and dorsalis pedis arteries. In non-diabetic subjects the pressure is similar in the two arteries, but in diabetics occlusion of one of the calf arteries might produce marked differences in the measured pressures. The pressure may be expressed in absolute terms or as the ratio of ankle/brachial pressure. The latter is the more common measurement and is sometimes called the Pressure Index (PI) which in normal subjects is ≥ 0.9. Placing appropriate cuffs at other levels in the leg may allow estimates of the pressure in the vessels of the upper part of the calf and the thigh, but these estimates bear a less certain relationship to intravascular pressure than measurements made at the ankle and their use in this way is not recommended.

How may this measurement be applied to the assessment of diabetics with foot lesions? In non-diabetics the level of the pressure index is a very valuable guide to the severity of the ischaemia and the prognosis in a particular patient. For example a PI of greater than 0.5 means that arterial reconstruction is not necessary. If the PI is less than 0.25 in a patient with ischaemic rest pain, lumbar sympathectomy is unlikely to be of benefit and unless reconstruction can be performed it is likely that amputation will be required.

There is, however, one serious qualification which must be remembered with diabetic patients. If the artery wall is calcified it may not be compressed when the occlusion cuff is inflated. This means that a distal flow signal will still be audible although the cuff pressure is well above systolic pressure. In these circumstances the ankle pressure measurement is of no value. It is not always possible to predict this eventuality but an experienced observer will be alerted when he hears an abnormal flow signal in an artery in which the pressure is measured at or near normal levels. There is little data on the frequency with which this occurs. It is difficult to predict if an artery will be compressible even if calcification is seen radiologically. Carter (1973) found that in 4/5 limbs with extensive calcification, the indirectly measured pressure was > 10 mmHg higher than the pressure measured directly and Gibbons et al (1979) found indirectly measured pressures of > 200 mmHg in 22 of 150 patients in their report.

The measurement of the ankle pressure is an important part of the assessment of these patients because it gives a more sensitive and objective guide to the blood supply to the foot than does palpation of ankle pulses. This method has been less successful than expected when used to predict healing of foot lesions or amputation wounds.

Healing of ulcers.   Carter (1973) suggested that healing was unlikely if the ankle systolic pressure was <55 mmHg. Above this level almost all non-diabetics would heal the lesion but amputation was necessary in 14 of 66 diabetics with pressures ≥55 mmHg. Raines et al (1976) stated empirically that healing was unlikely if the ankle pressure was <55 mmHg in a non-diabetic and <80 mmHg in a diabetic patient. It is said that on average the ankle pressure is higher in diabetics than in non-diabetics with lesions but this probably reflects the role of neuropathy and infection in the diabetic subjects. Arterial calcification would also tend to produce this result.

Healing of amputations.   Similar controversy exists over the role of these measurements in predicting the healing of amputation wounds. The most recent report from a centre with a large experience in the surgery of these patients (Gibbons et al 1979) found that for foot amputations a low ankle pressure (<70 mmHg) occurred as frequently in those whose amputations healed as in those in whom amputation failed. In the same report an ankle pressure of <70 mmHg occurred in 22 of 48 below-knee amputations (BKA) which healed successfully. Several reports have indicated that the level of the ankle systolic pressure is a useful predictor of healing of BKA. Barnes et al (1976) and Pollock and Ernst (1980) have both reported that healing is likely if the ankle pressure is at least 70 mm mercury. However healing will occur in some patients with lower ankle pressures so that using this criterion to exclude the possibility of a BKA will result in the performance of a larger number of higher amputations which are more disabling. The use of other methods which have a better predictive ability will be discussed below. The evidence suggests that Doppler pressure measurements are only moderately useful in predicting the healing of ulcers and amputations. Despite these limitations they may define groups of patients in whom, on the one hand, healing is to be confidently expected or, on the other hand, healing will be unlikely.

Mercury strain gauge

The pulse detector with this apparatus consists of a thin silastic tube filled with mercury which makes contact with copper wires at each end of the column. This gauge is placed around a digit or the limb. With each heart beat there is a small pulse in the tissues and this causes elongation of the gauge. With the change in length there is a proportional change in the electrical resistance of the column of mercury and this can be detected using a Wheatstone bridge or other appropriate circuit. The output can be led to a chart recorder. The blood pressure can be measured in two ways. Using an a.c. circuit the cuff pressure at which the pulsation returns can be recorded as the systolic pressure. Alternatively, using a d.c. circuit, systolic pressure can be recorded as the cuff pressure at which the volume of the part begins to increase. The pressures measured using the two techniques are closely related to each other and to the pressure obtained with the Doppler ultrasound method. The equipment is available as a package (e.g. Plethysmograph SP2, Medimatic, Copenhagen) or the components (e.g. Parks Plethysmograph, Beaverton, Oregon, U.S.A.) can be attached to a recorder of the user's choice.

A cuff placed above the ankle will allow the measurement of the systolic blood pressure at that level and the applications of this information have been discussed. If a cuff is placed around the base of a toe with a strain gauge distal to it, pressure can also be measured in the toe. This method, although not widely used, has a number of important applications:

a. Classification of patient. A toe systolic pressure of ≤20 mm mercury will be found in more than 70% of patients with rest pain or ischaemic ulcers but in less than 20% of patients who present with intermittent claudication (Tønnesen et al 1980).

b. Development of ulcers in diabetics. Diabetic patients have a higher pressure gradient between toe and ankle than non-diabetics. The highest gradients i.e. the lowest toe pressures, are found in patients with ulcers or gangrene of the foot (Faris 1975). This probably relates to the finding of proliferative intimal changes and occlusion of digital and metatarsal arteries.

c. Prediction of healing of ulcers or gangrene. If the toe pressure remains less than 20 mm mercury, the chances of healing a lesion of the foot are less than 10%. If the toe pressure is greater than 30 mm mercury healing can be confidently expected following local treatment (Holstein and Lassen 1980, & Fig. 9.5). A rise in the pressure following arterial reconstruction will permit local healing if the pressure rises to a level greater than 30 mm mercury. These results provide a much clearer discrimination than has been obtained from other methods of segmental pressure measurement.

Pulse volume recorder

This represents a modern version of the oscillometer which was one of the earliest instruments to be used in the assessment of patients with vascular disease. In its present form it consists of a series of sphygmomanometer cuffs which are placed around the leg at several levels. The cuffs are inflated to subdiastolic levels and

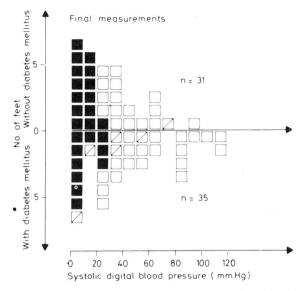

Fig. 9.5 Effect of toe systolic pressure on the healing of lesions of the foot. Closed squares — healing, square with diagonal line — healing following local amputation, open squares — major amputation. (From Holstein and Lassen 1980)

the pressure changes transmitted to them from the underlying arteries can be recorded. The equipment is available as a package and is widely used in vascular laboratories in the U.S.A. (Raines et al 1976). It is used to make qualitative assessments of the arterial pulsations and as a pulse detector for the measurement of segmental blood pressure. In diabetics it has been used in association with Doppler measurements to predict healing of ulcers and the results of forefoot amputation, but as has already been pointed out the accuracy of this prediction is not high (Gibbons et al 1979). This method is perfectly satisfactory for the measurement of ankle blood pressure although it has been found empirically to be useful for other purposes.

Arteriography
The distribution of arterial disease in the leg of diabetics was described in Chapter 3. If it is considered that the foot is unlikely to survive without arterial reconstruction, arteriography will help to determine if reconstruction is feasible. The indications for arteriography are thus the same in diabetics as in non-diabetics. It should be performed only when a decision has been made that operation is necessary or desirable. This decision is frequently made on clinical grounds in a patient with a history of rest pain or disabling claudication or with ischaemic ulcers or gangrene.

There is good evidence that angiography is ordered inappropriately in hospitals (Macpherson et al 1980). It should not be performed simply to determine the site and extent of arterial blockage in patients in whom the severity of the clinical features is not so great that non-operative treatment will be adequate or in whom a local amputation will be sufficient. Patients managed without arteriogram will include all diabetics in whom the ankle pulses are palpable or the ankle PI is ≥ 0.5

and most patients in whom the popliteal pulse is palpable. The latter group will only require arteriography if a graft to one of the calf vessels is being considered and this will be an unusual circumstance. The information required from an arteriogram, in addition to the site and extent of arterial occlusion, must include the state of the arteries above and below it. This usually means that the radiologist must display the arterial tree from the lower abdominal aorta to at least the mid calf level. It has been noted in Chapter 3 that distal occlusions are more common in diabetes so that frequently the radiologist will need to demonstrate the arteries down to the level of the ankle. This requirement lengthens the duration of the procedure and increases the discomfort to the patient. However the information thus gained is indispensable if surgical reconstruction to these distal vessels is being planned.

Several authors have reported the use of arteriography of the vessels of the foot. Cecile et al (1974) described patterns which they regarded as pathognomic of diabetes. The changes included hypervascularity and appearances which suggested microaneurysm formation. This technique has provided interesting parallels with vascular disease in other sites but is not useful in the management of patients.

Radioisotope methods

Isotope clearance

This is probably the best method for predicting the healing of below-the-knee amputations (BKA). The method as applied by Moore (1973) involves the intradermal injection of ^{133}Xenon dissolved in saline into the pretibial skin 10 cm below the tibial tuberosity. This level corresponds to the site of the anterior skin incision for a BKA (see page 119 for technique of amputation) and is the site at which ischaemic necrosis most commonly occurs. The rate of disappearance of the Xenon is dependent on the capillary blood flow and measurement of the rate of decrease of the radioactivity allows calculation of the blood flow. A critical level of flow of 2.6 ml/100 g/min reliably predicted healing in those limbs with greater flow and failure of healing if the flow was less than the critical level. The most recent report from this group (Malone 1979) indicates the results that can be obtained with careful assessment, good surgery and aggressive rehabilitation. In 133 patients (two-thirds of whom were diabetic) there were no postoperative deaths, 89% of amputations healed and all unilateral BKA patients were fitted with a prosthesis.

Skin blood pressure measurements

It has already been mentioned that skin blood flow varies in response to a variety of stimuli. It has been suggested that the blood pressure in the skin might not be so variable and thus a better indicator of the capacity of the skin circulation. Several methods of estimating the skin blood flow have been described. The best method again involves the study of ^{133}Xenon clearance from the skin (Lassen and Holstein 1974 & Fig. 9.6). In this technique external pressure, using a sphygmomanometer cuff, is applied over the injection site. The end point is reached when the pressure in the cuff is sufficiently high to just prevent further clearance of isotope from the skin. In normal subjects the pressure recorded is close to the di-

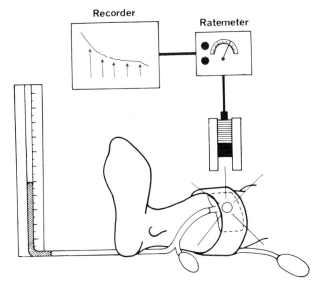

Fig. 9.6 Measurement of skin blood pressure. The end point is reached when the pressure in the cuff prevents further clearance of the isotope. The tracing recorded becomes horizontal. (From Lassen and Holstein 1974)

astolic blood pressure. The use of this method for the prediction of healing of major amputations has been reported (Holstein et al 1979a and c). If the skin perfusion pressure was greater than 30 mm mercury at the proposed site of the skin incision, major wound complications occurred in less than 10% of patients. However there was a very high frequency of wound complications if the skin perfusion pressure was below this value.

Other methods for assessing skin perfusion have been used. Holstein et al (1979b) used a photoelectric cell for recording the pressure which, when applied to the skin, caused blanching. This gave values similar to those obtained using the isotope clearance method. Using this method Holstein and Lassen (1980) found that healing of a foot lesion was certain if the pressure in the skin was recorded as 30 mm mercury or higher. Lee et al (1979) used similar apparatus to study the cutaneous circulation around bed sores and leg ulcers.

Chavatzas and Jamieson (1974) used the blanching of a histamine induced flare to indicate the level of the skin blood pressure. This technique used a transparent cuff and the end-point was the visually-determined blanching of the flare which is probably less precise than the isotopic method. The most recently used technique is the transcutaneous measurement of the oxygen tension in the skin (Matsen et al 1980). This apparatus has been used in paediatric centres for many years but has only recently been applied to the study of the circulation in the limbs. The principle is that the oxygen tension in the skin is a function of the skin blood supply. This sounds a promising idea and it is being intensively studied in a number of laboratories. It is too early to determine if the information provided will be useful clinically but the initial impression is that it is unlikely to provide information that will be valuable in discriminating between groups of patients.

Isotope perfusion scanning

This method involves the intra-arterial injection of radioactive material and the subsequent examination of the leg to determine the distribution of the isotope. The isotopically labelled particles are of a size that will be obstructed by a capillary bed. Two sorts of information can be gained for this study; each have been claimed to be useful in the management of patients.

Prediction of ulcer healing.   If the local blood supply is adequate to allow healing of an ulcer, there will be hyperaemia in the surrounding skin and a larger proportion of the injected isotope will accumulate in this area. This increased radioactivity can be measured. The most commonly used measurement has been the ratio of radioactivity in the surrounding skin to the radioactivity in the ulcer. A ratio has been used to try to minimize the importance of changes in skin blood flow which might result from such variables as anxiety, temperature changes and smoking. The critical value of the ratio has varied in different reports from 2.3– 3.5 (Siegel et al 1975; Johnson and Patten 1977). These authors suggest that the indications for use of this method include (a) delayed healing despite the presence of ankle pulses and (b) absent ankle pulses but an ankle pressure (using the Doppler technique) of more than 55 mm mercury. Patients with pressures lower than 50 mm mercury may be considered for reconstructive vascular surgery (see previous section).

Distribution of isotope within the leg.   The factors which determine the distribution of isotope to the tissues of the leg are poorly understood. It is important that the technique of injection should ensure adequate mixing of the isotope with the blood. It is clear that certain patterns of distribution can be recognized (Rhodes et al 1976). In the first, the isotope is distributed roughly in proportion to the muscle mass. If symptoms of ischaemia are present, this pattern is said to represent large vessel disease. In the second pattern, the isotope has a more patchy distribution and this is said to represent the presence of small vessel disease presumably involving arterioles and capillaries. These different patterns are easily demonstrated but their interpretation is open to question. In particular there is no clear explanation as to why the isotope should distribute preferentially to the skin if there is small vessel disease present, nor is there any histological evidence to support the interpretation given.

These isotope perfusion tests are easily applied in any centre with a nuclear medicine department. Their usefulness is not yet established although the technique to predict ulcer healing has the virtues of simplicity and an end-point which appears clear-cut. However in most cases it is likely that a trial of conservative therapy will be given before considering these extra tests and at the end of the trial period the chances of healing or progression will often be established. The study of the patterns of distribution of isotope to skin and muscle is not recommended until more data is provided concerning the mechanisms which produce the different patterns.

This section has described a variety of tests for assessing the severity of the vascular disease. The information gained is used to assess the severity of the vascular disease and thus to make predictions about the outcome, particularly in terms of spontaneous healing or healing following local surgery or amputation. The assessment of the severity of the arterial disease can be best made using one of the methods for measuring distal blood pressure. The Doppler method has the advantage that the apparatus is more portable but measurement of toe pressure provides additional useful information because it is probably the best predictor of local healing: if the pressure can be raised to greater than 30 mm mercury healing is likely. Radioisotopic methods also have a place in the armamentarium of a vascular laboratory. The presence of hyperaemia around an ulcer is a useful predictor of healing. However their greatest value is in the prediction of healing following major amputation and for this reason there is a strong case for their routine use.

The achievement of the aims outlined above is of very great potential benefit both to individual patients and to the community. The accurate prediction of prognosis would mean that unnecessary and futile operations could be avoided. This would be expected to reduce morbidity and mortality for individual patients. The overall benefit would be a reduction in the hospital stay for many patients and there are great economic benefits in achieving even a modest reduction in the time which these patients spend in hospital. For these reasons, the wider use of the tests discussed here is to be encouraged as are efforts to find more precise methods.

REFERENCES

Barnes R W, Shanik G D, Slaymaker E E 1976 An index of healing in below knee amputation: leg blood pressure by Doppler ultrasound. Surgery 79: 13–20
Carter S A 1973 The relationship of distal systolic pressure to healing of skin lesions in limbs with arterial occlusive disease, with special reference to diabetes mellitus. Scandinavian Journal of Clinical & Laboratory Investigation Supplement 128, 31: 239–243
Cecile J P, Descamps C, Guaquier A, Faille J C 1974 Diabetic foot arteriography. Journal of Cardiovascular Surgery (Torino) 15: 12–20
Chavatzas D, Jamieson C W 1974 A simple method for approximate measurement of skin blood pressure. Lancet 1: 711–712
Faris I 1975 Small and large vessel disease in the development of foot lesions in diabetics. Diabetologia 11: 249–253
Gibbons G W, Wheelock F C Jr, Siembieda C, Hoar C S Jr, Rowbotham J L, Persson A B 1979 Noninvasive prediction of amputation level in diabetic patients. Archives of Surgery 114: 1253–1257
Holstein P, Dovey H, Lassen N A 1979a Wound healing in above knee amputations in relation to skin perfusion pressure. Acta orthopaedica scandanavica 50: 59–66
Holstein P, Nielsen P E, Barras J-P 1979b Blood flow cessation at external pressure in the skin of normal human limbs. Photoelectric recordings compared to isotope washout and to local intra arterial blood pressure. Microvascular Research 17: 71–79
Holstein P, Sager P, Lassen N A 1979c Wound healing in below-knee amputations in relation to skin perfusion pressure. Acta orthopaedica scandanavica 50: 49–58
Holstein P, Lassen N A 1980 Healing of ulcers of the feet correlated with distal blood pressure measurements in occlusive arterial disease. Acta orthopaedica Scandanavica 51: 995–1006
Johnson W C, Patten D H 1977 Predictability of healing of ischemic leg ulcers by radioisotopic and Doppler ultrasonic examination. American Journal of Surgery 133: 485–489
Lassen N A, Holstein P 1974 Use of radioisotopes in assessment of distal blood flow and distal blood pressure in arterial insufficiency. Surgical Clinics of North America 54: 39–55
Lee B Y, Trainor F S, Kavner D, Cresologo J A, Shaw W W, Madden J L 1979 Assessment of the healing potentials of ulcers of the skin by photoplethysmography. Surgery Gynecology & Obstetrics 148: 232–239
Macpherson D S, James D C, Bell P R F 1980 Is aortography abused in lower-limb ischaemia? Lancet 2: 80–82
Malone J M, Moore W A, Goldstone J, Malone S J 1979 Therapeutic and economic impact of a modern amputation program. Annals of Surgery 189: 798–802

Matsen F A III, Whyss C R, Pedegana L R, Krugmire R B, Simmons C W, King R V, Burgess E M 1980 Transcutaneous oxygen tension measurements in peripheral vascular disease. Surgery Gynecology & Obstetrics 150: 525–528

Moore W S 1973 Determination of amputation level. Archives of Surgery 107: 798–802

Pollock S B Jr, Ernst C B 1980 Use of Doppler pressure measurements in predicting success in amputation of the leg. American Journal of Surgery 140: 103–106

Raines J K, Darling R C, Buth J, Brewster D C, Austen W G 1976 Vascular laboratory criteria for the management of peripheral vascular disease of the lower extremities. Surgery 79: 21–29

Rhodes B A, Bader P, Stoltz K, White R I, Siegel M E 1976 Assessment of peripheral vascular disease in patients with diabetes. Two case studies. Diabetes 25: 307–314

Siegel M E. Giargiana F A, Rhodes B A, Williams G M, Wagner H N Jr 1975 Perfusion of ischemic ulcers of the extremity. Archives of Surgery 110:265–268

Tønnesen K H, Noer I, Paaske W, Sager P H 1980 Classification of peripheral occlusive arterial disease based on symptoms, signs and distal blood pressure measurement. Acta Chirurgica Scandanavica 146: 101–104

Williams H T, Hutchinson K J, Brown G D 1974 Gangrene of the feet in diabetics. Archives of Surgery 108: 609–611

Yao S T 1970 Haemodynamic studies in peripheral arterial disease. British Journal of Surgery 57: 761–766

10

Management

This chapter describes the management of patients with infections, ulcers and gangrene. Their severity ranges from a minor area of skin loss resulting from wearing a new pair of shoes, to large areas of necrosis and spreading infection. The common factor among them all is a break in the integrity of the skin. Once this occurs the most important barrier to infection has been lost and thus the risks to the patient are greatly increased. It cannot be emphasized often enough that the best management of these lesions is to prevent them developing. In Chapter 7 the routine care that should be given to all diabetics was described and the treatment of early lesions was discussed. Detailed plans of management for more serious lesions will be given in this chapter.

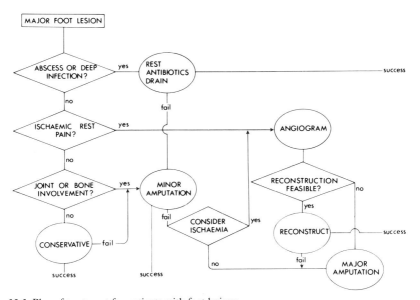

Fig. 10.1 Plan of treatment for patients with foot lesions.

The flow chart illustrated (Fig. 10.1) shows a plan which can be followed. In order to preserve clarity in the figure not all the possible combinations of events are shown, but the major pathways are suggested. The indications for operative treatment are:

1. abscess or deep infection
2. severe ischaemia

3. osteomyelitis or suppurative arthritis
4. spreading anaerobic sepsis. This condition is not illustrated in the chart because of its rarity. However if it is present it requires urgent treatment, usually a major amputation.

The methods of treatment considered are:

a. Conservative treatment
b. Drainage of an abscess
c. Minor amputation
d. Arterial reconstruction
e. Major amputation

The techniques for performing the various operations are described later in the chapter.

Abscess or deep infection

The clinical features have been discussed on page 77. Minor infections can be treated with rest and antibiotics. However great care should be taken not to overlook an abscess because it cannot be cured by antibiotic therapy alone and local spread will result in continuing loss of tissue. For this reason early drainage of an abscess of the foot is important. The diagnosis of an abscess deep in the foot may be difficult but satisfactory healing will not occur unless deep infections are detacted and drained. If there is tendon exposed in the base of an ulcer or there is evidence of osteomyelitis on a radiograph of the foot, the presence of a deep infection can be safely assumed. Adequate drainage in these circumstances will require more than an incision and the ray amputation (p. 104) is often employed.

During the 24–48 hours before operation is undertaken the control of the diabetes can be improved and antibiotic therapy will reduce the cellulitis and decrease the chance of the infection spreading following operation.

Severe anaerobic infection is fortunately a rare event but it is the most serious outcome of infection in a foot. These patients have extending muscle necrosis which progresses rapidly up the leg. There may be swelling and tenderness in the calf and it will be apparent that the patient is seriously ill with fever, tachycardia and leucocytosis, and often septic shock. The commonest setting is in a patient who has undergone a partial foot amputation. In these circumstances, after restoration of the circulating blood volume and administration of large doses of antibiotics, a major amputation must be undertaken urgently. The possible use of hyperbaric oxygen therapy has been discussed on page 43. Figure 10.2 shows a suggested plan for the management of infection.

Ischaemic rest pain

The characteristics have been described on page 84. If this symptom is present it means that there is an occlusion of the large blood vessels in the limb above the ankle.

If arterial reconstruction is not feasible either because of the general condition of the patient, the extent of the gangrene or, most commonly, the anatomy of the arterial obstruction, major amputation (see p. 119) will be the likely outcome. The same result is likely following failure of a reconstruction. The absence of rest pain does not mean that arterial disease is absent because neuropathy may keep even a severely ischaemic foot free from pain. In these patients decision

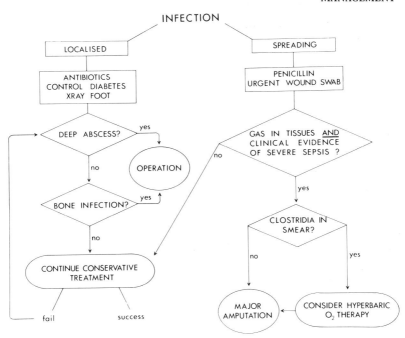

Fig. 10.2 Flow-chart for the management of a patient with an infected foot.

making is much more difficult and disagreements with the suggested plan are more likely. The possible outcomes are discussed below. A minor amputation may be performed following a successful reconstruction in order to remove dead tissue.

Bone or joint infection

Infection which has involved a bone or joint is unlikely to resolve without excision of the affected area. The diagnosis can be made by either gentle probing of a sinus or demonstrating exudation when a joint is moved. The radiological signs of infection (p. 82) may be difficult to distinguish from neuropathic joint change (see p. 35), but if there is an ulcer over a joint which shows these changes, it is likely that the joint is infected. These patients do not always undergo operation. In a foot with a normal blood supply a more conservative approach using plaster of Paris immobilization may be advocated and, certainly in patients with leprosy, can be used successfully. It would be regarded as more conventional in diabetic patients to excise the affected area, often using the ray amputation.

Conservative treatment

If none of the features described above is present, conservative treatment may be continued while improvement is occurring. The reasons for failure of conservative treatment are the presence of an abscess, joint or bone involvement, ischaemia and failure to alleviate mechanical causes. It is essential at all stages to consider the possibility of an abscess in the foot. If this has been excluded the next step is commonly to perform a local amputation in an attempt to secure healing. Failure of a local amputation is likely to be due to either infection or ischaemia. The former will require further local surgery, but the latter will require a successful arterial reconstruction if the foot is to be saved. There are two groups of major lesions which are often treated conservatively.

Neuropathic ulcers

Details of the treatment have been given on page 65. This may be continued as long as there are no signs of deep abscess or osteomyelitis. In many patients the regimen can be continued for months or years and may be repeated if an ulcer recurs. Such a policy requires meticulous supervision and this is very time-consuming. In addition, there is always the risk of infection which might result in the loss of more tissue. If an ulcer fails to heal or recurs several times it may be decided to attempt a cure by means of surgery. However, this should not be regarded as the easy solution because:
1. the operation carries risks of infection and failure of healing
2. the period of reduced mobility in or out of hospital will involve 4–6 weeks
3. careful follow-up is still required to prevent further lesions.

Ischaemia without rest pain

The plan outlined in Figure 10.1 has deliberately taken a conservative approach to the management of patients in this group. The alternative approach is to consider arterial surgery in all patients in whom there is significant ischaemia i.e. with absent ankle pulses. Neither approach is without hazard. The most serious objection to the latter approach is that even in the absence of ankle pulses, wounds and ulcers may heal if the collateral circulation is adequate and therefore arterial surgery is not needed. This successful result occurred in 89% of Sizer and Wheelock's (1972) series following local amputation. In these circumstances it is a serious error to submit the patient not only to angiography, which is painful and carries small but definite risks of arterial occlusion or embolism, but also to the dangers and discomforts of a major operation (see page 114 for an estimate of the risks of these operations). The other plan is to treat small areas of gangrene conservatively or with local amputation. The risk of this is that the blood supply will be inadequate and the consequent failure of healing enhances the chances of developing spreading anaerobic sepsis. This can be minimized with careful supervision and prophylactic antibiotic therapy. Failure of local surgery means that the patient must have a successful arterial reconstruction if the foot is to be saved (Fig. 10.3). However the chances of successful reconstruction are unaltered by the previous local amputation although it is true that a greater loss of tissue is probable. The crucial assessment required is of the adequacy of the collateral circulation: if this could be made with confidence, the difficulties discussed in the preceding paragraph would cease to exist. The use of the tests described in chapter 9 can reduce the uncertainty. However as noted in that section, none of the tests is entirely satisfactory and the importance of the problem justifies the continuing search for better methods.

NON-OPERATIVE TREATMENT

The principles involved are rest and antibiotic therapy. A number of methods have been advocated in an attempt to avoid major amputation in patients with se-

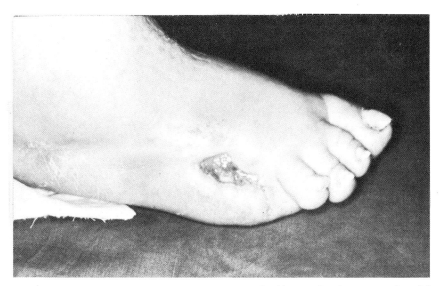

Fig. 10.3 Healing of foot following a successful femoropopliteal bypass. Previous amputation of the fifth toe had resulted in gangrene extending onto the dorsum of the foot

vere ischaemia who are unsuitable for arterial surgery and these will be discussed briefly.

Rest

The aim of treatment is to avoid the mechanical factors which precipitated the episode and thus to allow healing to occur. Strict rest in hospital is not often used, largely for economic and social reasons. In immobile or bed-ridden patients great care must be taken to avoid new pressure areas developing so that both feet must be carefully protected. The achievement of this simple aim requires meticulous nursing care. The heels and the malleoli are the most vulnerable areas. A cradle will usually be placed in the bed to keep the bedclothes off the feet.

A number of methods of protecting the feet are used. Some are more effective than others. Boots made of sheepskin or synthetic material with similar properties are probably the best. They have the advantage that they can be easily removed to allow inspection of the foot. They should be made to cover as much of the foot as possible and if they are fixed by a strap across the dorsum of the foot, great care must be taken that the strap is not too tight because pressure lesions can develop there, too. If these boots are not available a bulky cotton wool dressing kept in place by a crepe bandage is probably the next best choice. The wool must be thick over the heels and malleoli and the bandage must not be too tight. This is an important part of the postoperative dressings (see p. 106). Devices which use slings attached to bedframes are not recommended. They make nursing care more difficult, reduce the patient's mobility in the bed and, worst of all, are very difficult to keep properly positioned.

If the patient is allowed to continue walking an effort should be made to allow a period of rest during the day. The benefits can be explained to the patient in simple mechanical terms, e.g. if walking is reduced by 20% then this will similarly reduce the stresses which caused the ulcer.

The other measures which might be taken to relieve stresses on the foot have been described in Chapter 7. These include care of toenails (p. 63), removal of hyperkeratotic skin (p. 65) and provision of splints and footwear (p. 66). All these important steps must be continued whether the patient is to be managed as an outpatient or if hospital care is required.

Antibiotic therapy
The indications for antibiotic therapy and suggested regimens have been given in Chapter 5 (see p. 44).

Non-operative treatment of gangrene
Many patients with gangrene due to ischaemia are considered unsuitable for arterial surgery. There are three major groups:

1. elderly patients with gangrenous patches on the foot (see p. 73)
2. patients who present with extensive gangrene so that no useful part of the foot can be saved. This includes about one quarter of all patients presenting with severe ischaemia
3. patients with rest pain but with arterial disease which is not amenable to reconstruction.

The first group are frequently managed conservatively, attempting to avoid further trauma and giving antibiotic therapy for infection. For the other groups the pathway indicated in Figure 10.1 leads to major amputation and this is the most frequent outcome. A number of methods have been used to try to avoid this result in the third group of patients.

Correction of polycythaemia and thrombocythaemia
About 25% of patients with polycythaemia rubra vera present with arterial complications. This, of course, applies to non-diabetics as well as diabetics. Similarly, thrombocythaemic patients may present with areas of skin necrosis frequently on digits. The commonest cause of polycythaemia in patients with leg ischaemia is chronic hypoxia due to raised carboxyhaemoglobin levels associated with smoking.

In all three groups of patients further necrosis can be prevented by treating the blood disorder. If the patient is being considered for arterial reconstructive surgery it is very important to treat the polycythaemia and thrombocythaemia before operation because operation on patients with a high haemoglobin or platelet count has a very high complication rate (Bouhoutsos et al 1974).

Hypertension
The induction of moderate hypertension, e.g. by use of mineralocorticoid drugs, can produce an improvement in distal blood pressure and flow which can be of clinical benefit (Lassen et al 1968). The side effects, especially fluid retention, are potentially serious for patients with impaired myocardial function but with careful supervision complications can be avoided.

Haemodilution
This has been studied particularly from the view of reducing the use of blood transfusion during operation. Haemodilution produces an increase in cardiac out-

put and peripheral vasodilatation while maintaining oxygen delivery to the tissues (Shah et al 1980). On the basis of the observed reduction in blood viscosity, it has been suggested that chronic haemodilution might improve peripheral blood flow and thus promote the healing of ischaemic areas. There has been one report claiming benefit (Rieger et al 1979).

Prostaglandins

These drugs have complex actions on the circulatory system. They cause a reduction in peripheral resistance and an increase in cutaneous blood flow. Patients with severe ischaemia have been successfully treated using intra-arterial infusion of prostaglandins (Szczeklik et al 1979; Sethi et al 1980). In view of the lack of benefit obtained from vasodilator drugs, the benefits for this regimen might have resulted from the inhibition of platelet activity produced by the drug.

Solcoseryl

This substance is a protein-free extract of calf blood which has been demonstrated to facilitate healing of lesions in patients with advanced atherosclerosis. It has been shown to be effective in avoiding amputations in patients with severe ischaemia (Charlesworth et al 1975). Its mode of action is unknown but in experimental situations it has been shown to increase oxygen uptake by tissue and this may be the reason for the improvement seen.

The preceding paragraphs have described reports which provided reasonable evidence that the method advocated spared the patient a major amputation. In achieving this they have been of significant benefit. Despite this potential, the methods are not widely used. There are several reasons for this, including the need for intra-arterial infusion, the potential side effects, e.g. from induced hypertension and the limited availability of the drugs, e.g. prostaglandins. In addition there is the doubt about the duration of relief: does the patient really gain if amputation is only postponed for 3 months? Despite these objections, the potential benefits are great and the search for better methods of treatment will continue.

No mention has been made of the use of vasodilator drugs. It is considered that they have no place in the management of these patients, with or without diabetes. There has never been satisfactory evidence of benefit from their use, and there are strong theoretical arguments against them. It can be shown that the small vessels in severely ischaemic areas are already dilated and the only possible effect of vasodilator drugs is to shunt blood away from the affected areas by dilating normal vascular beds.

SURGERY

Preoperative management

Control diabetes.   Good control of the diabetes will not be attained until infection has been drained but ketosis must be corrected and hyperglycaemia should be reduced, usually by insulin injections (see Appendix for details).

Control infection.   A period of antibiotic therapy is essential for about 24–48 hours prior to drainage of an infected foot, except in the presence of spreading anaerobic infection when operation is needed within hours of diagnosis. Preoperative antibiotic therapy will decrease the surrounding cellulitis and may reduce the chances of spread of septicaemia, but if there is a deep abscess indicated by swelling of the foot and separation of the toes antibiotics are never sufficient treatment. The choice of antibiotics is discussed on page 44.

LOCAL AMPUTATIONS

A wide variety of local amputations may be performed in order to preserve a useful foot. The extent of the operation will be governed primarily by the extent and spread of the necrosis and infection, and only secondarily by consideration of the appearance of the foot. The use of eponyms to describe these procedures has been kept to a minimum in this account. This is because improvization and opportunism, rather than detailed knowledge of numerous procedures, are important attributes of the surgeon confronted with these difficult problems.

It has long been an axiom that the first amputation should be the last. While this certainly applies to major amputations, it is an underlying theme of this section that, because there is no precise way of estimating the adequacy of the blood supply, one attempt at a local amputation is often justified. However, as soon as it becomes clear that healing will not occur (and this is often at the time of the first change of the wound dressings), urgent steps should be taken to determine if arterial reconstruction is possible. If it is not, further delay in performing the major amputation only reduces the chances of rehabilitation of the patient. In particular repeated attempts at successively higher amputations of the foot are to be deprecated.

The principles governing local amputations are:

a. Exploration and excision must be thorough but gentle. Remaining tissues must never be handled by anything harder than the surgeon's fingers.

b. Never use a tourniquet.

c. Infected areas must be opened widely. There is no place for small incisions of fluctuant areas and the insertion of drain tubes through the foot. There is usually deep infection, e.g. in bone, which cannot be drained adequately without wide incision and excision of devitalised tissue. The apparent gains from small incisions will be outweighed by the losses from persistently draining sinuses and re-exploration for recurrent infection, and if the blood supply is adequate, a large incision will heal just as well as a small one.

d. Protect the other foot at all times. It may be the only one the patient will have.

Ray amputation

This operation, which removes a toe and the distal half of a metatarsal shaft, is considered by many to be the most useful of the local amputations. It has the advantages of providing excellent drainage of the deep parts of the foot and also removing the prominent metatarsal head beneath an ulcer. The postoperative management, which is described in detail, can be applied to patients having the other operations discussed in this section.

Indications

Infection involving a single metatarso-phalangeal joint arising from a trophic ulcer

Infection in the deep flexor tendon sheaths, e.g. arising from an infected gangrenous toe

Technique

It is essential that the operation provides adequate drainage of ALL infected areas of the foot. Collections of pus commonly form on the dorsum of the foot over the heads of the metatarsals. In the sole of the foot the infection tends to track medial to the heel pad, towards the tip of the medial malleolus.

The incision (Fig. 10.4) encircles the base of the toe and extends proximally into the sole. It may pass through the ulcer which need not be excised although minimal trimming of the thick skin in the area of the ulcer may be carried out. The toe is disarticulated at the metatarsophalangeal joint. The distal part of the plantar incision is deepened to the metatarsal shaft which is freed from its soft tissue attachment by dissection with a scalpel and a raspatory. The dorsal incision may be extended proximally if there is a collection on the dorsum of the foot. This will also facilitate mobilization of the metatarsal shaft. The bone is divided with bone cutters at approximately the middle of the shaft. Further proximal dissection is difficult and damages the transverse arch.

This procedure results in a wound which, when viewed from the plantar aspect, is deepest distally and gradually becomes more superficial proximally (Fig. 10.5 and 10.6). This allows blood and exudate to discharge onto the dressings and does not permit the infected material to track proximally into the foot. The length of the incision is thus determined by the need to plan the wound according to these requirements, and to drain the most proximal areas of infection. The skin wound should extend 1–2 cm proximal to the level of bone section. The wound is packed with gauze wet with a non-irritant solution, e.g. saline. The whole foot including the heel is then wrapped in a bulky cotton wool dressing which is held in place by crepe bandages. The toes should be left exposed so that they can be inspected and palpated.

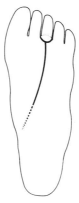

Fig. 10.4 Ray amputation. Incision.

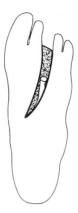

Fig. 10.5 Ray amputation. Appearance at end of operation.

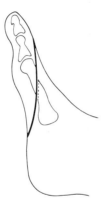

Fig. 10.6 Ray amputation. Shelving appearance of wound seen from the side.

Postoperative care

The principle of protecting the feet from further trauma must continue to guide the management in the post-operative period. A cradle in the foot of the bed keeps the bedclothes clear and allows easy inspection. Narcotic analgesics are seldom required because of the degree of neuropathy that is often present. Severe pain is an urgent indication to inspect the wound. The five day course of antibiotic therapy should be completed. Fever should resolve within 36 hours of operation and any recrudescence is an indication to examine the wound. The wound should also be inspected if there is any suspicion of a deep infection in the leg. This may be suggested by fever, pain in the leg (this pain need not be severe), and redness and swelling of the lower leg.

In the absence of any of these complications the dressings should be removed about the 5th postoperative day. This is best carried out in the operating theatre because there is often the need for further excision of small areas of necrotic tissue. If the facilities in the ward are adequate it is permissible to perform the first dressing in the ward where minor areas of necrosis may be excised. This careful revision of the wound is extremely important and may need to be repeated several times before the condition of the wound is satisfactory. Healing can occur despite the presence of small areas of necrosis but these provide foci from which recurrent abscesses may develop. These often present several weeks after the patient has been discharged from hospital and, in addition to the inconvenience of repeating the whole process of drainage and review, there will be more loss of tissue.

When the wound is free of necrotic tissue, it is sufficient to insert the edge of a gauze swab into the depths of the wound in order to keep the edges apart. This dressing can be changed daily in the ward until the wound is clean and granulating, when the edges can be allowed to fall together. There should be no hesitation in returning the patient to the operating theatre for further revision of the wound or excision of dead tissue should this be necessary. After about 14 days the bulk of the dressings may be reduced and the patient permitted to walk, with supervision, to the bathroom. The wound will take several weeks for complete healing but good cosmetic and functional results are likely.

This account of the operation and postoperative care has been given with what may seem to be obsessive attention to detail. No apology is made for this approach because failure to exercise sufficient care may result in loss of the foot, and this should be regarded as great a disaster as, for example, the loss of a limb that has been operated on for intermittent claudication.

Toe amputations, single toe

Indications
Gangrene of one digit in the absence of rest pain
Perforating ulcer of the interphalangeal joint of the great toe

Technique
This varies with the digit involved. For the great toe the incision is made around the base of the toe and extended 2–3 cm proximally along the medial border of the foot. The tendons and soft tissues are divided and the toe disarticulated through the metatarsophalangeal joint. If there is any doubt about the cleanliness of the wound it should be left open for closure at a later date but if the wound is apparently free of infection, the skin may be closed with adhesive paper tapes (e.g. Steristrips). Prolonged delay in closing the wound may result in retraction of the skin flaps and closure may be impossible without removing part of the metatarsal head. However, if the wound is closed too early infection may result and this causes further loss of tissue. If there is adequate skin, it is not necessary to excise the head of the first metatarsal because preserving it leaves an important weight-bearing structure. If the degree of skin involvement means that the head of the metatarsal cannot be preserved, the shaft of the bone should be divided obliquely to provide a rounded contour to the medial side of the foot.

Postoperatively the patient need not as a routine be returned to the operating theatre for inspection of the wound, and walking may be allowed at about the end of the second week.

For the other toes it is usual to (a) incise the skin at the junction of living and dead tissue, (b) carefully strip the soft tissues from the bone, and (c) divide the bone through the base of the proximal phalanx or disarticulate at the metatarsophalangeal joint.

When carried out in this conventional manner the operation may fail because, when the patient is supine, the most dependent part of the wound into which exudate will drain has ready access to the deep tissues of the foot by way of the flexor tendon sheath which has been opened. These patients may present with a deep infection of the foot several weeks after apparently satisfactory healing. To avoid this complication the skin incision should be extended 1–2 cm proximally on either the plantar or dorsal aspect of the foot, so that the wound can drain freely (see detailed description of ray amputation). This advice is contrary to the axiom that potentially ischaemic tissues are not incised. However in these patients infection, not ischaemia, is the greater problem. The wound should be managed as described for amputation of the great toe.

All (remaining) toes

The clawed toes on a neuropathic foot have a negligible role in walking but they are vulnerable to minor trauma and these episodes, if followed by infection, may cause major morbidity. If there is no doubt about the adequacy of the blood supply of the foot, amputation of healthy toes is sometimes justified. The patient is usually worried about the assault on his body image and the patient (and often his attending physician) need reassurance that walking will be unaffected. It has been demonstrated that in normal subjects loads equivalent to about 30% of the bodyweight are carried by the toes in the period just before the foot is lifted from the ground. In diabetics with neuropathy less than 10% of the bodyweight is borne by the toes during this phase of walking (see Chapter 6). This, combined with the observation of patients who have had all toes amputated (or even a transmetatarsal amputation), allows the patient to be reassured that his walking and balance will not be noticeably different than before operation.

The operation is advised in the following circumstances:

a. Repeated abrasion and ulceration of the dorsum of the toes that cannot be prevented by the provision of adequate footwear.

b. The need to amputate (for other reasons) the great or fourth toe. Removal of the great toe makes the second toe particularly liable to trauma and subsequent removal of the second toe makes the remaining toes successively vulnerable. Removal of the fourth toe leaves a fifth toe which is both vulnerable and useless. Incisions are made around the base of the toes and for a short distance down the medial and lateral sides of the foot (Fig. 10.7). The toes are disarticulated at the metatarsophalangeal joints and the wound closed with adhesive paper tapes. The final appearance is illustrated in Figure 10.8

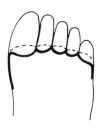

Fig. 10.7 Incisions for toe amputations. The medial and lateral extensions are necessary to allow dissection of the bases of the phalanges without vigorous retraction of the flaps.

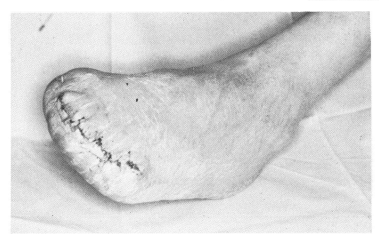

Fig. 10.8 Toe amputation. Final appearance.

Transmetatarsal amputation

This is the classic local amputation for diabetics and the technique and results have been reported extensively by McKittrick et al (1949), and more recently by Wheelock (1961).

Indications

Gangrene involving more than one toe

Persistent or recurrent plantar ulcer (Fig. 10.9)

The conditions for the successful performance of the operation have been stated by Wheelock (1961) to be:

1. Gangrene must be localised to a toe or toes and must not extend onto the foot.

2. Infection must be localised.

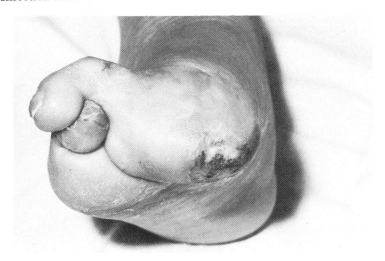

Fig. 10.9 Indications for transmetatarsal amputation. This patient has an ulcer over the first metatarsal head, a previous ray amputation and useless toes.

3. There must be no rest pain.
4. The venous filling time must be not greater than 20 seconds.
5. Dependent rubor must be absent or minimal.

Technique

The incision across the dorsum of the foot is at the level of the middle of the metatarsal shafts (Figs. 10.10, 10.11). The plantar incision is at the base of the toes. These two incisions are joined along the medial and lateral borders of the foot. The plantar flap is dissected to contain as much soft tissue as possible and the dorsal incision is carried down to bone. The metatarsals are divided at the level of the dorsal incision. This can be carried out by an amputation saw, taking great care not to damage the skin flaps. Alternatively, the bones can be divided individually by a Gigli saw or bone cutters (the latter method may splinter the bones). Visible tendons are removed from the plantar flap which is then folded to approximate the dorsal incision. The wound is closed with adhesive paper tapes and produces a dorsally placed scar.

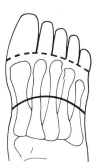

Fig. 10.10 Transmetatarsal amputation. Dorsal view of incisions

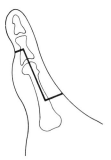

Fig. 10.11 Transmetatarsal amputation. Medial view of incisions

Discussion

The surgeon must often choose between a ray and a transmetatarsal amputation. The former is preferred if there is a deep abscess in the foot because it provides better drainage. The ray amputation has the disadvantage that it reduces the number of weight-bearing metatarsal heads from 5 to 4, while the transmetatarsal amputation preserves five metatarsals and may produce a better load distribution. However shortening the foot may produce greater stresses as discussed on page 55. The greatest problems in making the choice between the two operations occur when a patient is being considered for operation for persistent or recurrent plantar ulceration. If a single ray is involved, it is the author's preference to perform a ray amputation. Some prefer a transmetatarsal amputation if the first ray is involved because of the belief that due to the high load carried by the first metatarsal, there will be an unacceptable risk of recurrence if this bone is removed. My own view is that neither the clinical results nor the evidence from the studies of the mechanics of the foot strongly support this view. If two rays are involved, a transmetatarsal amputation is preferred because of a high risk of recurrence if only three weight-bearing metatarsals remain (see Fig. 6.8). The indications and technique described by Wheelock for this extremely useful operation have produced excellent results but this may have been at the price of excluding from consideration many patients who had more extensive disease. It is conceded that broadening the indications will result in the inclusion of patients in whom a higher failure rate is to be expected and this will tend to discredit the procedure. However denying this procedure to these patients will result in the loss of many feet, when in many cases useful parts could be saved. It is in situations like this that difficult decisions arise. In general, if ischaemic rest pain is absent, it is reasonable to attempt a local amputation, and a variety of these 'ad hoc' procedures can be performed. The two major determinants of success are the care with which the operation is performed and the adequacy of the blood supply. Two specific examples will be discussed:

a. If infection or ulceration involves two rays transmetatarsal amputation is preferred to ray amputation. However the presence of infection deep in the foot is a contraindication to transmetatarsal amputation. In these circumstances, transmetatarsal amputation with delayed closure of the wound is an acceptable procedure.

b. An important group of patients who may be helped by these operations are those who have presented with gangrene of the foot and in whom a successful arterial reconstruction has been performed. This discussion therefore applies as much to non-diabetic patients as to diabetics. Conventional transmetatarsal amputation may be contraindicated because the necrosis often extends beyond the toes. In these cases, amputations may be performed more proximally in the foot, e.g. by disarticulating metatarsal from tarsal bones. As much plantar skin as possible should be preserved. Infected wounds should be left open and defects may be closed secondarily, sometimes by split skin grafts. By rigid application of the principles outlined and by meticulous wound care many gratifying results can be obtained (Fig. 10.12).

It can be argued that a formal Syme's amputation could be preferable in these circumstances. This may have the advantage of more rapid healing which results from successful direct closure of the wound but preservation of the tarsal bones allows a normal shoe to be worn and this is a considerable long-term advantage which should not be discarded lightly.

Syme's amputation

For the reasons given above it is the author's preference to perform an amputation which will preserve as much of the tissues of the foot as possible. However, some surgeons argue that the durability of the stump and the rapidity of healing

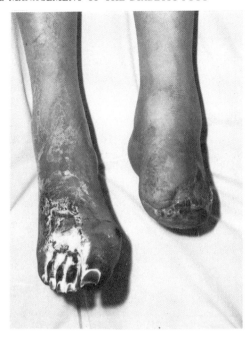

Fig. 10.12 The left foot shows the result obtained following femoropopliteal bypass, local amputation and skin graft for gangrene of the toes. An almost identical lesion developed in the right foot 12 months afterwards. This was treated similarly and the foot healed

still give this operation a useful place. In these circumstances, the operation would be indicated in a foot with gangrene which is too extensive to allow the safe performance of a transmetatarsal amputation, and in which the blood supply is judged to be sufficient to allow healing.

The plantar incision is made from the tip of the lateral malleolus to a point 2 cm below the tip of the medial malleolus. The dorsal incision joins the ends of the plantar incision and divides the structures which run anterior to the ankle joint. On the medial side, the flexor tendons and plantar vessels and nerves are divided and laterally, the peroneal tendons are encountered and divided. The ankle joint is entered by dividing its anterior ligament and the collateral ligaments are cut. These manoeuvres allow progressive plantar flexion of the foot. The posterior ligament is divided from within the ankle joint and the calcaneum is dissected from the heel flap. During this part of the procedure great care must be taken to protect the branches of the posterior tibial artery which are closely applied to the posterior ligament because the viability of the flap depends on their preservation. The malleoli are sectioned at, or just above, the level of the ankle joint ensuring that the cut is perpendicular to the long axis of the bones. The heel flap is brought forward and sutured in position.

The operation results in shortening of the limb by about 5 cms. The length and bulbous end of the stump make it difficult to fit a foot prosthesis although some form of 'elephant-boot' appliance may give very satisfactory functional results and there are other prostheses designed to accommodate this stump.

THE DIABETIC AND ARTERIAL SURGERY

The whole range of procedures which may be performed on non-diabetics can be carried out successfully on diabetics. For detailed accounts of the procedures and the techniques for their performance, a textbook on arterial surgery should be consulted. This section is concerned with arterial surgery for disease affecting the leg in diabetics.

One of the major problems in the management of diabetic patients has been to assess the role of arterial surgery. There have been two major difficulties in this area. The first is the view that diabetics fare poorly after arterial surgery so that the possibility of arterial reconstruction is frequently not considered. However, there are many reports which indicate that the results of performing arterial surgery on diabetics are only marginally inferior to the results obtained in non-diabetics. As outlined in Chapter 3, the characteristic pattern of arterial disease in a diabetic is a relative sparing of the aorta and iliac arteries and an increase in atherosclerotic occlusions in the arteries of the calf. Severe disease of the calf vessels often precludes reconstructive surgery (for exceptions see below) and the recognition of this pattern led to the view that diabetic patients were unsuitable for arterial reconstruction. It is true that there will be diabetic patients in whom arterial surgery cannot be performed but this also applies to non-diabetics although the proportion of patients with inoperable disease is greater among diabetics. The second major problem is the failure to recognize that, in a diabetic, gangrene may be treatable by local surgery without arterial reconstruction even if the axial arteries are obstructed. This has been discussed earlier in this chapter (page 100).

Indications for arterial surgery

These are the same in the diabetic as in the non-diabetic limb viz:
    intermittent claudication
    threatened loss of limb

Intermittent claudication

The diabetic patient with intermittent claudication should be considered for reconstruction according to the same criteria applied to the non-diabetic. If the claudication is severe enough to endanger employment or seriously interfere with domestic or leisure activities and the patient is unable to live within the limitations imposed by the claudication then surgery should be considered. The pain should have been stable for at least three months, or worsening. This is because there is a tendency for claudication of recent onset to improve as collateral vessels enlarge with the result that, after the concern at the initial development of the pain, the patient becomes able to live with the symptoms by adjusting his daily routines. The ability to walk 100 metres might represent a severe disability to one patient but might be easily tolerated by another of more sedentary habit. Another step which should be taken is to urge the patient to stop smoking. This may have two important effects. First, the progress of the vascular degeneration may be slowed and second, there is clear evidence that the chances of an arterial reconstruction remaining patent are higher if the patient has stopped smoking (Myers et al 1978).

The decision of whether to offer the patient an operation is also influenced by knowledge of the natural history of the disease, treated or untreated. The patient must be reassured that the symptom of claudication does not carry with it a high risk of eventual loss of limb and this knowledge often markedly increases the capacity of the patient to tolerate the pain. The attendants must also remember that there is a high (25–30%) risk that the patient will die of vascular disease in other areas, e.g. brain, heart or kidneys, within 5 years. The likely results of operation also influence the decision. Aorto-iliac surgery when successfully performed has a good (about 80%) long term patency. However, there is a significant mortality (1–5%) and this should be remembered before offering the patient an operation for a condition which does not directly threaten his life. Femoro-popliteal bypass surgery is safer (operative mortality about 1%) but is less effective in the long term. Many reports now suggest that the number of grafts patent 5 years after operation is of the order of 50–60% and these results are leading many surgeons to the view that femoropopliteal bypass should only be performed infrequently for the indication of intermittent claudication. The conservative view is that operation for claudication should be delayed as long as possible because, in the event of failure of the bypass, the patient may be worse off and there is then only a slim chance of restoring the situation if the saphenous vein has been used already. The more aggressive approach is that the patient should be given the opportunity to enjoy what is left of a limited life-expectancy. Whichever view is taken, it must be remembered that a successful reconstruction is not the end of the patient's problems.

Once the decision has been made to consider surgery then, and only then, should angiography be performed. It should not be ordered until it has been decided that arterial surgery will be performed if the anatomy is favourable (see p. 91).

Threatened loss of limb
The generally conservative approach outlined above is not suitable for patients in whom the survival of the limb is threatened. In these patients a major amputation will be necessary unless the arterial supply to the foot can be improved. The clearest indications for action exist in patients with ischaemic rest pain in the foot. Gangrene may or may not be present. This group of patients should be considered in the same way as non-diabetics. Arteriography should be performed to determine if arterial reconstruction is feasible. If reconstruction is not possible lumbar sympathectomy (page 118) may be considered in an attempt to delay the need for amputation, although this is only worthwhile considering if the skin is intact. More difficult decisions arise in patients when neuropathy coexists. These patients often have gangrenous patches over the heels and other pressure areas or non-healing ulcers which are painless. Many of the patients are elderly and frail and in the absence of pain or spreading infection no treatment is necessary. The risk taken when following this advice is that an aggressive infection may occur and the spread of the infection may result in loss of the limb (or even the life) of the patient. Against this must be weighed the risk of performing major surgery. Local areas of gangrene which are well demarcated ('dry gangrene') may be allowed to separate or be gently amputated.

A common and important group of patients are those in whom there is ulceration or gangrene which is not healing with conservative treatment and there is evidence of impairment of the blood supply to the foot. It is assumed that any infection has been adequately drained. In these patients a local amputation may be considered despite serious doubts about the adequacy of the blood supply to the foot. If rest pain is present angiography should be performed with a view to carrying out an arterial reconstruction, preferably at the same time as the amputation. In the absence of rest pain and in the absence of any simple test which will allow the outcome to be predicted with confidence (see Chapter 9), the course most often chosen will be to perform the local amputation. If it becomes apparent at the time the wound is inspected postoperatively that healing will not occur, angiography and successful reconstruction will be necessary if part of the foot is to be preserved. Once it has been decided to perform a local amputation, angiography is not necessary until it is established that healing will not occur.

If the gangrene is extending and if there is a prospect of the patient regaining mobility and it is believed that ischaemia is contributing significantly to the condition, arterial reconstruction should be considered and angiography performed.

Types of operations
The surgery carried out will depend on the extent of the arterial occlusion demonstrated on the arteriogram. The criteria are that there must be an adequate pressure above the area to be reconstructed and there must be patent vessels distal to the reconstruction so that the increased blood flow can be distributed to the peripheral tissues. It is this latter condition which may not be satisfied if there is extensive occlusion of the arteries of the calf. The patterns of disease encountered are:

Aorto-iliac stenosis or occlusion
To fulfil the first criterion given above, namely that there must be an adequate flow of blood into the reconstructed segment, means that aorto-iliac stenosis or occlusion must be corrected before femoral artery occlusion is treated. The two techniques commonly used are insertion of a bypass graft (usually made of dacron) from the aorta to each femoral artery (aorto-femoral bypass) or local disobliteration of the areas of narrowing or occlusion (thrombo-endarterectomy). The choice of operation will depend on the experience of the surgeon and the extent of the disease; bypass being preferred if there is extensive disease and endarterectomy if the disease appears more localized, e.g. to one common iliac artery. Disease localized to the external iliac artery is particularly favourable to endarterectomy.

Surgery involving operating on the abdominal aorta is dangerous. Any technical error is likely to require the transfusion of at least 1 litre of blood and, in addition, clamping the aorta causes a temporary impairment of renal function. To this must be added the cardiopulmonary effects of a major operation. For these reasons alternative approaches to the management of aorto-iliac stenosis and occlusion have been developed. Two major options are available. If the disease is confined to one iliac system a graft may be inserted from the femoral artery on the less affected side to the opposite femoral artery. This operation, femorofemoral crossover or bypass, carries a low risk and has a good long term patency. The graft, which may be either vein or synthetic material, is commonly placed in the subcutaneous tissue across the pubis and its patency can be checked easily. Because of its safety it is often used in frail patients. The alternative approach is to use the axillary artery as the donor vessel and connect it with the femoral artery via a long tube of Dacron which is placed subcutaneously over the lateral thoracic wall. This operation, axillofemoral bypass, is also safe but has the disadvantage that the use of a long prosthesis increases the chances of infection and occlusion. It has been suggested that the patency rate can be improved if the lower end of the graft is connected to a femoral crossover graft so that the blood flow through the long decending limb is increased and thrombosis is less likely to occur. This is a reasonable alternative operation in patients unfit for aortofemoral bypass.

Femoral artery occlusion
The commonest lesion affecting the blood supply to the leg is an atherosclerotic occlusion near the point where the femoral artery passes through the hiatus in the adductor magnus muscle, close to the shaft of the femur. Occlusion at this site commonly results in thrombosis of the femoral artery up to the next major branch which is the profunda femoris artery. Some propagation of the thrombus occurs distally but the popliteal artery usually remains patent because of the flow around the knee through the collateral vessels which enter the popliteal artery. Stenosis of the profunda femoris artery is present in 20–30% of patients with femoral artery obstruction. The profunda femoris artery supplies the thigh muscles and anastomoses via its terminal branches with the branches of the popliteal artery around the knee joint. The system of anastomoses may be so good that the patient is unaware of a femoral artery obstruction. Atheroma affecting the profunda femoris artery frequently involves only the first 1–2 cm and removal of this stenosing atheromatous material, (profundaplasty), can improve the blood supply to the limb so that more distal reconstruction is unnecessary. This procedure has the further advantage that it only requires a short groin incision and can, if necessary, be performed using local analgesia. The commonest procedure used to bypass obstruction of the femoral artery is a reversed saphenous vein graft from the femoral artery above to the popliteal artery below (femoropopliteal bypass). If the long saphenous vein is not available and the limb will be lost if reconstruction cannot be performed, there are a number of alternative procedures including the use of a synthetic tube but these grafts do not remain patent for as long as vein grafts.

In patients with symptoms of intermittent claudication, extensive disease of the calf vessels is regarded as a contraindication to operation. This is because the high fixed resistance of the distal arterial lesions will limit the blood flow through the graft and predispose to occlusion. In patients in whom the survival of the limb is threatened, a less favourable situation may be accepted. Fig. 10.13 shows the operative arteriogram obtained at the completion of a femoropopliteal bypass. There is no major vessel connected to the patent popliteal artery. Despite this severe disease the operation was followed by healing of a foot ulcer and the graft was still patent twelve months after operation. Femoropopliteal bypass may be attempted if there is a 3 or more centimetre long segment of popliteal artery patent and if a major amputation is the alternative procedure. Frequently there is no usable pop-

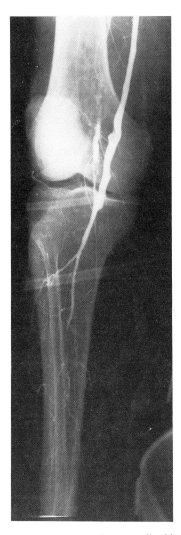

Fig. 10.13 Operative arteriogram at completion of a femoropopliteal bypass graft in a patient with severe disease of the calf arteries

liteal artery and a bypass to one of the tibial vessels is the only possible procedure. Femoropopliteal bypass has a similar prognosis in diabetics and nondiabetics (Stipa and Wheelock 1971; Barner et al 1974; Cutler et al 1976).

Femorotibial reconstruction

In recent years techniques have been developed to allow bypass grafting as far distally as the ankle. These procedures, which should only be performed if the viability of the limb is threatened, can be carried out with reasonable success and may last for periods of several years. Functionally there are three terminal branches of the popliteal artery: the anterior tibial, posterior tibial and peroneal arteries. The peroneal artery ends on the lateral and posterior surface of the calcaneum but its perforating branch, which pierces the interosseus membrane 5 cm above the ankle joint and ends on the dorsum of the foot, may occasionally take the place of the dorsalis pedis artery. Any one of the three terminal branches of the popliteal artery may carry sufficient blood to allow the foot to survive and may be the only possible site for insertion of a bypass graft if the popliteal artery is occluded. The principles of these operations are similar to those for standard femoropopliteal bypass but magnification is commonly used when carrying out the lower anastomosis. These operations can result in initial limb salvage in about half the patients (Reichle et al 1979). The initial success was less in diabetics (46% compared with 61% in non-diabetics), but the long term results were similar in both groups.

Lumbar sympathectomy

Removal of the lower part of the lumbar sympathetic chain removes the vasoconstrictor fibres to the skin of the foot. Within 24 hours of operation the foot becomes warm and dry: findings which give satisfaction to both surgeon and patient. However, close investigation suggests that these benefits are at best transient and at worst illusory. The blood flow to the foot increases by about 5 times shortly after sympathectomy but this increase is not maintained so that after 2–3 weeks the blood flow is about twice its preoperative value. There is no doubt, however, that many patients improve symptomatically following operation, but it is usually not possible to tell if this benefit is the result of operation or of the natural tendency to develop collateral pathways. In addition it can be demonstrated that the majority of the increased blood flow is through channels which act as arteriovenous anastomoses. These vessels bypass the capillary network so that the blood flowing through them is of no nutritional value to the tissue.

Another argument is the one used against the exhibition of vasodilator drugs. The vessels in a severely ischaemic area are already dilated, presumably under the influence of local metabolites which are the most potent stimuli of local vasodilatation. Under these circumstances removal of vasoconstrictor tone is likely to have the effect of lowering the resistance to flow through relatively normal vascular beds and thereby shunt blood away from the ischaemic areas: an effect opposite to that which is desired. In diabetic subjects there is an additional argument against sympathectomy because the effects of the neuropathy may have been to produce degeneration of the sympathetic fibres, and it can be argued that sympathectomy should only be considered in diabetics if vasoconstrictor tone can be demonstrated (see p. 30 for tests which might be used).

Despite these objections, there may be some patients in whom lumbar sympathectomy may be of benefit:

1. Patients with ischaemic rest pain who have too much calf vessel disease to allow reconstruction, and in whom the skin of the foot is intact. These are the patients who on conventional clinical grounds, are most likely to benefit. If the ankle PI (see p. 87) is less than 0.25 the operation is futile. If ulcers or gangrene are present the chances of a clinically successful result are much reduced.

2. As an adjunct to reconstructive surgery. There is some evidence that the probability of an arterial graft remaining patent is proportional to the volume of blood flowing through it. Lumbar sympathectomy performed at the time of reconstruction will increase the flow through the graft during the critical first few days of its life, and this may increase the chances of continued patency.

In performing the operation the aim is to denervate the vessels of the foot. This can be achieved by removing the 4th lumbar ganglion and short lengths of the adjacent sympathetic chain. It is no longer considered necessary to perform an extensive removal of the sympathetic chain between the renal and iliac vessels as was formerly taught.

MAJOR AMPUTATIONS

The aim of the measures discussed in the preceding sections of this book has been to preserve the legs and feet and avoid amputation. However in many patients the state of the limb makes no other course feasible. Even at this stage it is important to maintain a hopeful outlook. Although the overall results of amputation are not good, there are few more grateful patients than those relieved of the constant pain of an ischaemic limb.

The technique of these operations and rehabilitation postoperatively, do not differ in diabetics and non-diabetics and the reader is referred to other works (e.g. Little 1975) for details.

Below-the-knee amputation (BKA)

This very important and useful operation has regained favour in the last 10 years. If healing is successful there is a good chance that the previously mobile patient will walk again. With modern prostheses the patient can be provided with a limb which is held in place only by a strap around the knee and this gives the least possible inconvenience to the patient. The disadvantage of the procedure is that with the incision more distally placed in the limb, healing is less certain and most series have shown that the healing of a BKA is about 10% poorer than for higher amputations. The need to undergo a major reamputation is very serious for the patient: the mortality is of the order of 20% and there are the deleterious effects of a prolonged stay in hospital. If major amputation is necessary, most surgeons will try to perform a BKA in a previously mobile patient. The techniques to predict healing of amputations have been described in Chapter 9, and their wider use might improve the results. Patients who are bedridden or whose mobility is limited by frailty present different problems. In these patients the greater certainty of healing of a higher amputation is usually accepted. The major requirement of the limb is then to provide stability when seated and the ability to turn over when in bed and these aims can be achieved by an amputation performed at or just above the knee joint. There is a further disadvantage of a BKA in these patients. Flexor contracture of the knee joint is likely to occur and this provides another deformity to be coped with by the nursing staff. In these patients the BKA offers no advantages which counter the disadvantages described.

Technique

A variety of techniques are available and that using a long posterior musculocutaneous flap will be described. This is favoured because of the empirical observations, later supported by skin blood pressure studies, that the pretibial skin has a worse blood supply than the skin over the back of the calf. As a result ischaemic necrosis of the skin occurs most often at the distal edge of the anterior flap.

The skin incisions are marked out. The anterior incision is horizontally placed

10 cm below the tibial tuberosity and extends from the fibula laterally, half-way around the limb. From the ends of this mark, lines are drawn 10–12 cm distally in the long axis of the limb and the distal limits of these marks are joined transversely.

Much of the operation is carried out from the front of the limb. The anterior incision is carried through superficial and deep fascia. The anterior crural muscles are divided and the anterior tibial vessels which lie close to the interosseus membrane are divided and, if necessary, ligated. The muscles surrounding the fibula are divided and the fibula cut with a Gigli Saw at or 1 cm proximal to the intended line of section of the tibia. The posterior flap is now raised. At its distal limit it will divide the proximal part of the tendo calcaneus, and more proximally it includes the gastrocnemius muscle. The next step is the division of the tibia. The periosteum is elevated 1 cm proximal to the intended line of section and a bevel is cut at about 45° through the anterior 1 cm of the tibia. Note that this is the only dissection performed beneath the anterior flap. The division of the tibia is completed by a transverse saw cut. The lower leg and foot are now attached only by the deep posterior muscles of the calf. These are divided with a scalpel or amputation knife and the limb is removed. Bleeding from the cut ends of venous sinuses in the gastrocnemius muscle is usually more prominent than bleeding from the posterior tibial and peroneal vessels. Haemostasis is secured by clamping and ligating bleeding vessels. The posterior flap is now folded forwards over the tibia and its alignment inspected. It may be shortened if it has been cut too long. Dense collagenous tissue (tendon), which has a poor blood supply, may be excised from the distal part of the flap. If too much of the gastrocnemius muscle bulk has been retained, part of the muscle may be excised but the amount removed should be the minimum necessary to allow the posterior flap to be approximated to the anterior flap without tension. The deep fascia of the flaps may be sutured with chromic catgut sutures and the skin is closed with fine interrupted silk or nylon sutures or, preferably, with adhesive paper tapes. The difference in the lengths of the perimeter of the flaps often results in small 'dog ears' at each end. On no account should they be trimmed because this involves incisions into the flaps and impairs their blood supply. Remodelling of the wound will result in the dog ears being inconspicuous by the time the prosthesis is fitted. Haemostasis should be sufficiently good that a drain tube is unnecessary. The wound is covered with gauze and the stump wrapped in a bulky dressing of cotton wool held in place by crepe bandages.

Postoperative management
The patient may require occasional doses of narcotic analgesics but severe pain is an urgent indication for inspection of the wound. Cellulitis surrounding the wound requires that a swab be taken and immediately examined for micro-organisms, especially gram-positive bacilli. Symptoms of phantom pain, about which the patient should have been warned pre-operatively, are very common but not often severe. If the patient had experienced severe pain prior to operation, he will often consider that the pain from the wound is much less than the pain from the ischaemic foot. The most important part of the post-operative management is physiotherapy. From the first postoperative day the patient should be supervised

in performing quadriceps exercises and these must be continued energetically un-til the prosthesis is fitted. The quadriceps group of muscles is the major factor producing stability of the knee joint and the patient can be told quite honestly that the length of time before he walks again is dependent to a large degree on the strength of these muscles. The dressings are left undisturbed for 7 days provided that pain, fever or discharge do not indicate the need for earlier inspection of the wound. A lighter dressing can then be applied and attention directed to careful bandaging to minimize oedema formation in the stump. Sutures, if used, should remain for 14–21 days.

Variations

Design of the flaps. There are several possible alternative ways of designing the anterior flap. The flap may be made semi-circular and 5–6 cm long. At the other extreme, surgeons who are very worried about necrosis in this area may actually excise anterior tibial skin for 1–2 cm above the proposed line of bone section (call-ed a 'negative' anterior flap).

Guillotine amputations. If the amputation is being performed in the presence of sepsis, the operation may be planned so that the wounds are left open. The classic guillotine amputation divides all tissues at the one level. This has the ma-jor disadvantage that retraction of the skin causes a long delay in obtaining skin cover. A more practical alternative is the operation described by Silbert and advo-cated for use on diabetics by Catterall. In this operation, the skin and sub-cutaneous tissue are divided circumferentially at a level 5 cm below the site of bone section and folded back to permit division of the bones and remaining soft tissues. The skin flaps are then replaced and the cavity filled with Vaseline gauze. If the length of the flaps has been well judged, retraction of the skin flaps and healing will result in a soundly healed stump with a small stellate scar over its end. More recently Catterall (1978), who has an extensive experience of the treat-ment of diabetics, has preferred the long posterior flap technique described earlier.

Complications

Necrosis. Death of the wound edges results in failure of healing and this is the most serious local complication of amputation. Infection may be a factor, but usually necrosis occurs because the local blood supply is inadequate to maintain the viability of the tissues. Tight sutures are an important cause and, although many experienced surgeons regularly suture amputation wounds, it is believed that the technique of wound closure using adhesive paper tapes is more likely to be 'fail-safe'. Necrosis of a few millimetres of the wound edge is compatible with successful healing, but if the greatest width of the necrotic area is greater than 1 cm a long delay in healing will be the best result and higher amputation may be necessary. If substantial areas of necrosis are present, they should be excised at the junction of living and dead tissues and secondary healing awaited.

Persistent pain in the wound is a bad prognostic sign. A wound which has an adequate blood supply and is adequately immobilized becomes much less painful after a few days. Persistent pain which is not due to infection suggests that the blood supply is inadequate and the wound may fail to heal. Absence of pain, however, does not guarantee success. In a severely neuropathic and ischaemic limb, a wound may fail to heal although pain has been minimal or absent. This sequence is more common following foot amputations than following BKA.

Infection. One of the important uses of prophylactic antibiotics has been the virtual elimination of gas gangrene in patients having major amputations. The proximity of the wound to a reservoir of organisms, viz. the anus, and the resistance of sporing organisms to skin disinfectants combined with the presence of relatively ischaemic muscle creates the ideal conditions for the establishment of an anaerobic infection. Penicillin is the agent of choice and should be given with the premedication, and for 24 hours after operation (see p. 44).

Ischaemia as a cause of wound pain has already been mentioned. Infection is another important cause. In the most serious cases when gas gangrene develops, there will be a thin exudate from the wound and rapidly spreading muscle tenderness in a seriously ill patient. If examination of a smear of the exudate reveals the presence of sporing organisms, then urgent treatment must be undertaken (see p. 43). Fortunately, this is now a very rare sequence of events. Mixed infection which may include staphylococci, anaerobic bacilli and intestinal gram-negative organisms are much more common. The presence of necrotic tissue is an important contributing factor to the establishment of these infections, and this is one of the reasons why meticulous operative technique is necessary. If pyogenic infection becomes established, it is treated using standard principles.

Haemorrhage. The formation of a haematoma in the wound will delay healing and predispose to infection. The best prevention is careful haemostasis in the wound: a drain tube does not compensate for untidy surgery. If a haematoma forms it should be evacuated by reopening a short length of the wound and rebandaging the stump firmly. Remember that bandages which are too tight cause ischaemia. Secondary haemorrhage was once a feared complication following amputation. This probably occurred following the amputation of limbs with a good blood supply, e.g. following trauma or infection. In performing a BKA the major arteries may often be divided without major bleeding occurring, so that secondary haemorrhage is a very uncommon event.

Later complications. The amputation stump remains a vulnerable area. An apparently healed wound may be split open, usually following a fall, several weeks after operation. In addition, progression of ischaemia may result in ischaemic rest pain and ischaemic necrosis of the stump. Ulcers developing from excessive pressure from a poorly fitting prosthesis are another important cause of morbidity. If flexion contraction is allowed to develop it usually means that the patient will never manage a below knee prosthesis. Serious difficulties such as those described will occur in about 25% of patients (Little et al 1974).

Higher amputations

If a BKA is considered inapplicable, or if it fails to heal, a higher amputation may be necessary. The operation chosen will depend on the preference of the surgeon, the chances of fitting a prosthesis and the extent of the arterial disease. The three operations most commonly performed are a through-knee disarticulation, a supracondylar (Gritti-Stokes) amputation and a mid-thigh amputation. The first two owe their successful healing to the anatomy of the collateral arteries which, in the area of the knee joint, are in the subcutaneous tissue. In addition both operations involve the division of only small amounts of muscle tissue which has the practical advantage of making haemostasis easier and the theoretical advantage of decreasing the chances of anaerobic sepsis. Further, both operations preserve maximum length of limb to facilitate the management of a bed-ridden patient. The major disadvantages of the operations relate to the difficulties in fitting a prosthesis. The length of the stump means that the knee joint of a prosthesis must be placed lower than on the intact side. In addition, the bulbous lower end of the femur following a through-knee operation is more difficult to accomodate. Difficulty in fixing the patella following a supracondylar amputation may also cause problems for the prosthetist. These difficulties can be overcome with modern prosthetic techniques and, particularly if it is believed that walking is unlikely, it is the author's preference to perform a through-knee or supracondylar amputation if a BKA is not feasible. If reamputation is needed following failure of a BKA, the proximity of the anterior skin incision to the area of ischaemia or necrosis usually means that a mid-thigh amputation will be necessary.

REHABILITATION

There are two major aims when considering a patient for possible amputation.

1. To produce healing by removing a painful and/or infected and therefore dangerous limb or part of a limb

2. To restore mobility

The achievement of the second aim begins preoperatively when the nature of the operation is discussed. While many patients would rather die than have a leg amputated, most will respond to a positive attitude on the part of their advisors who should emphasize the relief of pain, the removal of a dangerous or useless limb and the chances of walking again. An approximate timetable for the fitting of the prosthesis may be given. This will depend on local policies and the availability of limb-fitting facilities. In a patient having a BKA the importance of quadriceps function must be emphasized.

The greatest contribution to rehabilitation is made by the surgeon who carefully and meticulously performs the operation because a major factor delaying rehabilitation is problems with the amputation wound. It is following operation that the widest divergence in practices occurs. The conventional conservative approach has been to await healing of the wound and then refer the patient to a specialist in limb-fitting and rehabilitation who, often at another centre, undertakes the subsequent management. At the other extreme, all the amputations are performed by a single group of surgeons, immediate fitting of a prosthesis undertaken, and a co-ordinated programme of aggressive rehabilitation is begun. The results which can be achieved by this type of programme are shown by the report of Malone et al (1979) when half below knee amputees had a definitive prosthesis fitted by 32 days following operation. The only reservation held about these results is that they may have been a highly selected group of patients. However most surgeons would be happy to achieve these results, even if they were able to select their own patients! A major difference between the two approaches is the immediate fitting of the prosthesis which has the advantages that the wound is immobilized so that pain is less and healing is better; the stump does not become oedematous so that fitting a definitive prosthesis is easier and the patient can bear weight on the amputated limb within a few days of operation. These advantages may represent a considerable benefit for the patient. The reduction in pain and early mobility are good for morale and the maintenance of muscle power, and any resulting reduction in hospital stay is obviously beneficial.

The disadvantage is that necrosis and infection may not be detected until late because of the unwillingness of attendants to remove the rigid dressing and this may result in serious problems for the patient should these complications occur. In addition, the best results are likely to be obtained if there is a team which is regularly using the technique and which has adequate resources to function efficiently. An intermediate course is to use a prosthesis based on an air-filled splint as described by Little (1971). This device consists of a standard air-splint which is supported by a metal socket to which is attached a prosthetic foot. In the early post-operative period the air-splint provides support to the wound, subsequently it provides the socket which joins the limb to a temporary prosthesis. This method has the great advantage that the air-splint can be removed when necessary and reapplied easily.

There is a strong argument for forming a rehabilitation team to serve a large hospital or groups of hospitals. The evidence suggests that the money saved by such groups would pay the costs many times over and many more patients would be walking sooner.

PROGNOSIS

The outlook for groups of patients having major amputations is bad: the operative mortality is up to 10% and more than half the diabetic patients will be dead in two years (Finch et al 1980). Nor is there a favourable prognosis for the remaining limb. In about half the surviving patients a new lesion develops within 2 years and some of these require amputation (Goldner 1960; Brodie 1970). The results of rehabilitation of surviving patients are also poor: only about half become independently mobile or mobile beyond their own homes (Little et al 1974; Finch et al 1980).

REFERENCES

Barner H B, Kaminski D L, Codd J E, Kaiser G C, Willman, V L 1974 Haemodynamics of autogenous femoropopliteal bypass. Archives of Surgery 109: 291–293

Bouhoutsos J, Morris T, Chavatzas D, Martin P 1974 The influence of haemoglobin and platelet levels on the results of arterial surgery. British Journal of Surgery 61: 984–986

Brodie I A O D 1970 Lower limb amputation. British Journal of Hospital Medicine 4: 596–604

Catterall R C F 1978 in Diabetes and its management. Oakley W G, Pyke D A, Taylor K W, Oxford Blackwell Scientific Publications 3rd edn. p. 169

Charlesworth D, Harris P L, Palmer M K 1975 Intra-arterial infusion of Solcoseryl: a clinical trial of a method of treatment for pregangrene of the lower limb. British Journal of Surgery 62: 337–339

Cutler B S, Thompson J E, Kleinsasser L J, Hampel G J 1976 Autologous saphenous vein femoropopliteal bypass: Analysis of 298 cases. Surgery 79: 325–331

Finch D R A, MacDougall M, Tibbs D J, Morris P J 1980 Amputation for vascular disease: the experience of a peripheral vascular unit. British Journal of Surgery 67: 233–237

Goldner M G 1960 The fate of the second leg in the diabetic amputee. Diabetes 9: 100–103

Lassen N A, Larsen O A, Sørensen A W S, Hallböök T, Dahn I, Nilsén R, Westling H 1968 Conservative treatment of gangrene using mineralocorticoid-induced moderate hypertension. Lancet 1: 606–609

Little J M 1971 A pneumatic weight-bearing temporary prosthesis for below-knee amputees. Lancet 1: 271–273

Little J M 1975 Major amputations for vascular disease. Churchill Livingstone, Edinburgh

Little J M, Petritsi-Jones D, Kerr C 1974 Vascular amputees: a study in disappointment. Lancet 1: 793–795

McKittrick L S, McKittrick J B, Risley T S 1949 Transmetatarsal amputations for infection or gangrene in patients with diabetes mellitus. Annals of Surgery 130: 826–842

Malone J M, Moore W S, Goldstone J, Malone S J 1979 Therapeutic and economic impact of a modern amputation program. Annals of Surgery 189: 798–802

Myers K A, King R B, Scott D F, Johnson N, Morris P J 1978 The effect of smoking on the late patency of arterial reconstruction in the legs. British Journal of Surgery 65: 267–271

Reichle F A, Rankin K P, Tyson R R, Finestone A J, Shuman C R 1979 Long-term result of femoroinfrapopliteal bypass in diabetic patients with severe ischaemia of the lower extremity. American Journal of Surgery 137: 653–656

Rieger H, Köhler M, Schoop W, Schmid-Schönbein H, Roth F J, Leyhe A 1979 Haemodilution (HD) in patients with ischaemic skin ulcers. Klinische Wochenschrift 57: 1153–1161

Sethi G K, Scott S M, Takaro T 1980 Effect of intra-arterial infusion of PGE_1 in patients with severe ischaemia of lower extremity. Journal of Cardiovascular Surgery 21: 185–192

Shah D M, Prichard M N, Newell J C, Karmody A M, Scovill W A, Powers S R 1980 Increased cardiac output and oxygen transport after intraoperative isovolemic hemodilution. Archives of Surgery 115: 597–600

Sizer J S, Wheelock F C 1972 Digital amputations in diabetic patients. Surgery 72: 980–989

Stipa S, Wheelock F C 1971 A comparison of femoral artery grafts in diabetic and non-diabetic patients. American Journal of Surgery 121: 223–228

Szczeklik A, Nizankowski R, Skawinski S, Szczeklik J, Gluszko P, Gryglewski R J 1979 Successful treatment of advanced arteriosclerosis obliterans with prostacyclin. Lancet 1: 1111–1114

Wheelock F C 1961 Transmetatarsal amputation and arterial surgery in diabetic patients. New England Journal of Medicine 264: 316–320

Appendix
Perioperative management of diabetes

INTRODUCTION

In many patients admitted to hospital because of a foot lesion, the diabetes will be poorly controlled at the time of admission. Except in the most urgent circumstances, a patient should not be submitted to a general anaesthetic if diabetic ketosis is present. On the other hand, it is recognized that the pre-operative control of the diabetes will often be imperfect particularly if there is an abscess present. The aim of the management is to control the blood glucose as well as possible without causing intraoperative hypoglycaemia which may have devastating neurological effects; and to maintain nutrition so as to avoid the catabolic state characteristic of uncontrolled diabetes, since this would be an undesirable exaggeration of the normal metabolic response to surgery.

This brief account outlines the ways in which the diabetes might be managed during the perioperative period in patients undergoing the range of operations described in Chapter 10. At the outset it should be stated that there is often a conflict of interest in these cases. The management of the diabetes is facilitated if the operation is performed at a pre-determined hour, preferably in the morning. However, these patients often have heavily contaminated wounds and for this reason are placed at the end of the operating list in order to allow time for subsequent cleaning of the theatre and to minimise the risks for following patients.

If possible the control of the diabetes should be assessed by repeated estimations of the blood glucose concentration. The alternative — reliance on urinary glucose levels — has several disadvantages:

1. Control is retrospective because the urinary sugar reflects the blood concentration in the preceding hours.

2. If the renal threshold is not known, it is difficult to relate the urine sugar to blood sugar levels.

3. It may be difficult to obtain appropriately timed specimens without catheterization which carries risks of infection.

Fortunately it is now a relatively simple matter to obtain rapid bedside measurement of the blood glucose, using either a portable blood glucose analyzer or simple glucose oxidase-impregnated sticks yielding a colour reaction which can be measured either with a reflectance meter or visual comparison against a chart. The latter method, while semiquantitative, is of sufficient accuracy for monitoring diabetic control, and greatly simplifies the perioperative management of diabetes.

PREOPERATIVE MANAGEMENT

Insulin treated
The patient's usual insulin dose may be continued and supplementary regular insulin, 5–10 units depending on the blood sugar concentration, given at midday and evening if control has deteriorated. If, however, the patient has a large (> 50 units) insulin requirement or is severely hyperglycaemic or ketotic, then long or intermediate-acting insulin should not be used and regular insulin should be given 3–4 times daily, as follows:

a. patient eating normally — approximately ⅓ of previous total requirement before each meal with a dose adjustment for the blood sugar level, e.g. for patient on 30 units–

Blood glucose mmol/l	Insulin dose units
< 7	8
7–11	10
> 11	15

Such 'sliding scales' *must* be individualized and adjusted according to response, and insulin must not be omitted because the blood glucose is normal.

b. not eating normally — 5% dextrose, 1 litre every 8–12 hours, should be given continuously using a separate i.v. line. Insulin may then be given 6 hourly on a schedule similar to that outlined above. In any case, long-acting insulin should be reduced by 25% on the day prior to planned surgery.

Oral hypoglycaemics
Patients should be given insulin treatment unless the planned surgery is very minor and there is not likely to be any major change in food intake. The dose of insulin required is often between 10–20 units per day although as mentioned above, the requirement may be greater if there is a large septic focus. Oral hypoglycaemics may be continued in normal doses provided that the diabetes is well controlled.

DAY OF OPERATION

1. Insulin. Give half the daily requirement of both regular and intermediate-acting insulin. This will be half the patient's usual dose or if varying amounts have been given in the preceding days, half the estimated requirement for the day of operation.

2. Insert an intravenous infusion of 5% dextrose to run at the rate of 1 litre in 8 hours.

INTRAOPERATIVE

1. Continue i.v. dextrose 5% at rate of 1000 ml in 8 hours, again keeping the infusion separate from other lines which are used to replace intraoperative losses of fluid or blood.

2. During a long operation (> 2 hours), hypoglycaemia is unlikely, but glucose should be monitored hourly by the semiquantitative measuring-strip method.

3. If hypoglycaemia occurs dextrose 50% 10 ml may be given intravenously and repeated according to response. Avoid giving amounts in excess of those necessary to bring the blood glucose to a safe level (8–10 mmol/l).

POSTOPERATIVE

Day of operation

1. Insulin. Aim to give the remainder of the daily insulin requirement, which will be increased rather than decreased, in 2 doses: half immediately post-operatively and half 6 hours later. In most cases it will be convenient to continue 6–8 hourly administration of regular insulin on the same schedule outlined for preoperative use, aiming to keep the blood sugar in the range 3–11 mmol/l.

2. Nutrition. If oral feeding is possible, a normal calorie intake should be resumed as soon as possible. This may be given as liquid in the earliest periods. If oral feeding is not possible, continue the i.v. dextrose infusion.

Subsequent days

1. Insulin treated patients. If feeding is established and diabetic control not disturbed, the normal insulin dose may be resumed on the second postoperative day. Otherwise, divided doses of regular insulin should be continued along with blood glucose monitoring until the situation improves.

2. Patients on oral hypoglycaemics. Once oral feeding is established, the diabetes is well controlled, and the insulin requirement is not greater than 20 units per day, treatment with oral hypoglycaemic agents may be resumed.

THE PLACE OF INSULIN INFUSION

Where facilities exist, and particularly for severely uncontrolled patients, the use of continuous i.v. infusion of insulin is a powerful tool. It requires the facility for frequent — usually hourly — blood glucose measurement and should be confined to areas experienced in its use. Usually, blood glucose level can be maintained in the range 4–10 mmol/l by appropriate adjustment of the infusion rate according to the blood glucose level.

SUMMARY

The general principles for the management of these patients are:
1. Maintain carbohydrate nutrition throughout.
2. Maintain insulin availability at all times.
3. Avoid hypoglycaemia.

Index

Abscess of foot
  bacteriology, 43
  clinical features, 77
  treatment, 98
Amputation
  below the knee, 119
  complications, 121
  Gritti-Stokes, 122
  local, 104–112
  major, 119
  mid thigh, 122
  prediction of healing, 89, 92
  ray, 104
  rehabilitation, 123
  Syme's, 111
  through knee, 122
  transmetatarsal, 109
  toe(s), 107, 108
Anaerobic infection, *see* Infection anaerobic
Anatomy, 49
Angiography, 91
Ankle joint, 50
Ankle pressure index, 88
Antibiotic therapy, 43
Aortoiliac disease, 11
  surgery for, 115
Arches of foot, 49
Arterial surgery, 113–118
Arterial calcification, *see* Calcification of arteries
Arteries
  of calf, 11
  of foot, 13
Arterioles, *c.f.* Microangiopathy
  proliferative changes, 17
Atherosclerosis
  as cause of lesion, 5
  assessment, 83
  autopsy studies, 9
  diagnosis in limbs, 9, 87
  distribution, 11
  effects, 22
  mechanisms, 10
  occurrence, 9
Autonomic neuropathy, 29–33
  as factor in infection, 39
  cardiac effects, 31
  clinical features, 29

histology of, 27
  prognosis, 29
  tests of, 31
  vasomotor effects of, 29
Axillofemoral graft, 116

Bacteriology, 42
Blood flow measurement
  effect of arterial calcification, 14
  in early diabetes, 18
Blood lipids, 10
Blood pressure
  in legs, 87
  in skin, 92
Blood supply
  effects on inflammation, 39
Bones of foot
  infection, 82, 99
  neuropathic change, 35

Calcification of arteries, 14, 83
  effect on blood pressure
    measurement, 89
Callus
  formation, 49, 55
  removal, 62, 65
Capillary basement membrane thickening, 16
Capillary basement membrane permeability, 18, 39
Cardiac disease, 81
Care of foot, 60
Cellular response to inflammation, 40
Chemotaxis, 40
Chiropody, 62–66
Clawing of toes, 34, 86
Clostridium perfringens, 43
Collagen production, 41
Conservative treatment, 99
Control of diabetes
  assessment, 80
  effect on complications, 58
  effect on wound healing, 42
  perioperative, 126–128
Cranial nerve lesions, 29

Deformity of foot, 34
  footwear for, 66

Digital arteries, 13, 22
Disrupting forces, 47
Doppler ultrasound, 87
2, 3-DPG, 19

Education of patient, 60

Femoral artery occlusion, 11
   management, 116
Femoral crossover graft, 115
Femoropopliteal bypass, 116
Femorotibial bypass, 117
Fibrinolysis, 20
Footwear, 66
Forces under the foot, 51–55
   changes in diabetics, 55
   in presence of ulcer, 55
   normal pattern, 52
Forefoot, loads on, 52
Fungal infections, 42

Gait, phases of, 50
Gangrene
   clinical features, 72–74
   history, 2
   management, 114
   of toes, 72
   with infection, 74
Gangrenous patches, 73

Haemodilution, 102
Haemoglobin A_{Ic}, 19, 58
Harris mat, 52
Heart rate, beat-to-beat variation,
   31
Hyperbaric therapy, 43
Hyperglycaemia
   and vascular disease, 10, 14
   and infection, 41
Hyperinsulinism, 10
Hyperkeratosis, see Callus
Hypertension
   induced, 102
   occurrence, 10

Infection, c.f. Abscess
   anaerobic, 43, 78
   as cause of lesions, 5
   assessment of, 82, 98
   bone and joint, 99
   clinical features, 76
   non-clostridial 43, 78, 98
Inflammatory response
   abnormalities of, 39
Ingrowing toenail, 63
Insoles, 68
Instructions to patients, 60
Insulin
   and wound healing, 42
   history, 2
   perioperative, 126–128
Intermittent claudication, 22, 113

Ischaemia
   assessment, 83
   clinical features, 72
   management, 100
      c.f. Arterial surgery
Ischaemic
   necrosis, 47
   rest pain, 72, 83
Isometric exercise, 33
Isotopes, see Radioisotopes

Joints of foot
   Charcot, 35
   effects of neuropathy, 35
   infection, 82

Keratosis
   see Callus

Loads on foot
   see Forces under the foot
Lumbar sympathectomy, 118

Mechanics of foot, 48–55
Mercury strain gauge, 90
Metabolic causes of neuropathy, 26
Metatarsals, loads on, 54
Microangiopathy, 15–21
   aetiology, 18
   as cause of lesions, 5
   effects on foot, 22
   functional, 18
   hypoxia and, 18
   inflammation and, 39
   in muscle, 16
   in nerve, 16
   pathology, 16
   smoking and, 21
Monocyte function, 41
Mononeuropathy, 29
Muscles
   of calf, 50
   of foot, 34, 51

Nephropathy, 81
Nerve
   conduction, 27
   cranial, 29
Neuropathic
   joints, 35
   ulcers, see Ulcers, neuropathic
Neuropathy
   as cause of ulcer, 5
   assessment of, 86
   autonomic, see Autonomic neuropathy
   causes, metabolic, 26
   causes, vascular, 25
   clinical features, 27
   effects on foot, 33
   electrophysiological changes, 27
   history, 2
   mechanism of ulcer formation, 57

Neuropathy – *contd*
  mononeuropathy, 29
  pathology, 27
  somatic, 28

Onychogryphosis, 64
Osteomyelitis, 82, 99
Oxygen transport, 19

Penicillin, 45
Pes cavus, 49, 55
Phagocytosis, 40
Plantar fascia, 49
Plasma proteins, 20
Plastazote, 68
Plaster of Paris immobilization, 66
Platelet function, 10, 20
Plethysmography, 90
Polycythaemia, 102
Polymorphonuclear leucocytes, 40
Postoperative care, 106
Postural hypotension, 32
Precipitating factors, 6
Predisposing factors, 5
Preoperative management, 103
Pressure Index, 88
Pressure necrosis, 47
Profunda femoris artery
  profundaplasty, 116
  stenosis of, 11
Prostaglandins, 103
Prosthesis
  air splint, 124
  immediate fitting, 123
Pulse volume recorder, 90
Pulses, arterial, 84

Radioisotopes
  perfusion scanning, 94
  predict amputation healing, 92
  skin perfusion pressure, 92
Radiology of foot, 35, 82
Rehabilitation after amputation, 123
Renal function, 81
Repetitive stress, 48
Rest pain
  clinical features, 83
  treatment, 98
Retinopathy, 81

Shoes
  choice of, 61
  custom built, 67
  new, 48
  rocker shoe, 67
Skin
  blood pressure, 92
  response to pressure, 49
  temperature, 57, 85

Small artery occlusion
  definition, 8
  effects on foot, 22
  history, 2
Social factors, 62, 81
Solcoseryl, 103
Staphylococcus aureus, 38, 42
Stress fracture, 48
Surgery
  indications, 97
  perioperative management of diabetes, 126
  preoperative management, 103
Sweating, 30
Syme's amputation, 111
Sympathectomy, lumbar, 118

Tendon reflexes, 28
Thermography, 57
Threatened loss of limb, 114
  cf. Gangrene; Rest pain
Thrombocythaemia, 102
Toe
  amputation, 107, 108
  effects of neuropathy, 34
  loads carried, 54
  nails
    care of, 61
    ingrowing, 63
    lesions of, 63
  ulcers, 65, 76
Transmetatarsal amputation, 109
Trophic changes, 34

Ulcers, ischaemic, 73
Ulcers, neuropathic
  clinical features, 65, 75
  development, 57
  history, 2
  loads on, 55
  management, 65, 100
  on toes, 65, 76
  prediction of healing, 89, 94
Ultrasound
  measurement of blood pressure, 87

Valsalva manoeuvre, 32
Vascular disease
  and infection, 39
  as cause of foot lesions, 5, 22
  as cause of neuropathy, 25
Vasomotor neuropathy, 30

Walking
  causing repetitive stress, 48
  mechanics, 48
Windlass action of plantar fascia, 49, 55
Wound
  dressing, 101, 106
  infection, 38